Biomechanics of the Lower Extremity

Editor

JARROD SHAPIRO

CLINICS IN PODIATRIC MEDICINE AND SURGERY

www.podiatric.theclinics.com

Consulting Editor
THOMAS J. CHANG

January 2020 • Volume 37 • Number 1

ELSEVIER

1600 John F. Kennedy Boulevard • Suite 1800 • Philadelphia, Pennsylvania, 19103-2899

http://www.theclinics.com

CLINICS IN PODIATRIC MEDICINE AND SURGERY Volume 37, Number 1
January 2020 ISSN 0891-8422, ISBN-13: 978-0-323-71231-6

Editor: Lauren Boyle
Developmental Editor: Laura Kavanaugh

Clinics in Podiatric Medicine and Surgery (ISSN 0891-8422) is published quarterly by Elsevier Inc., 360 Park Avenue South, New York, NY 10010-1710. Months of issue are January, April, July, and October. Business and Editorial Offices: 1600 John F. Kennedy Blvd., Ste. 1800, Philadelphia, PA 19103-2899. Customer Service Office: 3251 Riverport Lane, Maryland Heights, MO 63043. Periodicals postage paid at New York, NY and additional mailing offices. Subscription prices are $304.00 per year for US individuals, $597.00 per year for US institutions, $100.00 per year for US students and residents, $382.00 per year for Canadian individuals, $721.00 for Canadian institutions, $457.00 for international individuals, $721.00 per year for international institutions, $100.00 per year for Canadian students/residents, and $220.00 per year for foreign students/residents. To receive student/resident rate, orders must be accompanied by name of affiliated institution, date of term, and the *signature* of program/residency coordinator on institution letterhead. Orders will be billed at individual rate until proof of status is received. Foreign air speed delivery is included in all *Clinics* subscription prices. All prices are subject to change without notice. POSTMASTER: Send address changes to *Clinics in Podiatric Medicine and Surgery*, Elsevier Health Sciences Division, Subscription Customer Service, 3251 Riverport Lane, Maryland Heights, MO 63043. **Customer Service: 1-800-654-2452 (US). From outside of the US, call 314-447-8871. Fax: 314-447-8029. E-mail: JournalsCustomerService-usa@elsevier.com (for print support); JournalsOnlineSupport-usa@elsevier.com (for online support).**

Reprints. For copies of 100 or more of articles in this publication, please contact the Commercial Reprints Department, Elsevier Inc., 360 Park Avenue South, New York, NY 10010-1710. Tel.: 212-633-3874; Fax: 212-633-3820; E-mail: reprints@elsevier.com.

Clinics in Podiatric Medicine and Surgery is covered in *MEDLINE/PubMed (Index Medicus)* and *EMBASE/Excerpta Medica.*

Contributors

CONSULTING EDITOR

THOMAS J. CHANG, DPM
Clinical Professor and Past Chairman, Department of Podiatric Surgery, California College of Podiatric Medicine, Faculty, The Podiatry Institute, Redwood Orthopedic Surgery Associates, Santa Rosa, California, USA

EDITOR

JARROD SHAPIRO, DPM, FACFAS, FACFAOM
Associate Professor, Western University of Health Sciences, College of Podiatric Medicine, Department of Podiatric Medicine, Surgery and Biomechanics, Program Director, Chino Valley Medical Center Podiatric Medicine and Surgery Residency with Rearfoot Reconstruction and Ankle Certificate, Pomona, California, USA

AUTHORS

JOSEPH H. ALTEPETER, DPM
Podiatry Resident, St. Vincent Hospital, Indianapolis, Indiana, USA

MARC A. BENARD, DPM
President and Co-Director, Baja Project for Crippled Children/Operation Footprint, Westlake Village, California, USA; Assistant Director, American Board of Podiatric Medicine, Hermosa Beach, California, USA; Clinical Associate Professor, Western University of Health Sciences, College of Podiatric Medicine, Pomona, California, USA

MELINDA A. BOWLBY, DPM, AACFAS
Attending Surgeon, Department of Orthopedics, Swedish Medical Center, Seattle, Washington, USA; Attending Surgeon, Department of Orthopedics, Providence Medical Center, Everett, Washington, USA

FRANCIS CHAN, DPM, AACFAS
Private Practice, Burnaby, British Columbia, Canada

TIMOTHY CHEUNG, MS, CPT
Student, Dr. William M. Scholl College of Podiatric Medicine, School of Graduate and Postdoctoral Studies, Rosalind Franklin University of Medicine and Science, North Chicago, Illinois, USA

JEFFREY C. CHRISTENSEN, DPM, FACFAS
Attending Surgeon, Department of Orthopedics, Swedish Medical Center, Seattle, Washington, USA; Attending Surgeon, Department of Orthopedics, Providence Medical Center, Everett, Washington, USA

DANA DAY, DPM
Clinical Instructor, Western University of Health Sciences, College of Podiatric Medicine, Pomona, California, USA; Resident, Chino Valley Medical Center, Chino, California, USA

PATRICK A. DEHEER, DPM FACFAS, FASPS, FACFAP, FFPM RCPS (Glasg)
Residency Director, Surgery, St. Vincent Hospital, Indianapolis, Indiana, USA; Staff
Surgeon, Surgery, Johnson Memorial Hospital, Franklin, Indiana, USA; Clinical Instructor
(Adjunct Track), Department of Podiatric Medicine and Radiology, Rosalind Franklin
University of Medicine and Science, North Chicago, Indiana, USA

ANKIT DESAI, DPM
Preceptor, Hoosier Foot and Ankle, Indianapolis, Indiana, USA

EVELYN G. HEIGH, DPM, AACFAS, FACFAOM
Guest Lecturer, Arizona School of Podiatric Medicine, Private Practice, Summit Medical
Group, Glendale, Arizona, USA

CHANDLER HUBBARD, DPM
PGY-2, Podiatry Resident, 2nd Year, Podiatric Medicine and Surgery with Rearfoot
Reconstruction and Ankle Certificate, Chino Valley Medical Center, Chino, California, USA

BETH JARRETT, DPM, FACFAOM, CPed
Associate Dean of Clerkship and Residency Placement, Associate Professor of Podiatric
Surgery and Applied Biomechanics, Dr. William M. Scholl College of Podiatric Medicine,
Rosalind Franklin University of Medicine and Science, North Chicago, Illinois, USA

BENJAMIN KAMEL, DPM
PGY-3, Chief Resident, PMSR/RRA Podiatric Residency, Chino Valley Medical Center,
Chino, California, USA

JONATHAN M. LABOVITZ, DPM, FACFAS
Associate Dean, Clinical Education and Graduate Services, Professor of Podiatric
Medicine, Surgery and Biomechanics, Western University of Health Sciences, College of
Podiatric Medicine, Pomona, California, USA

ELIZABETH OH, BS, CPT
Student, Western University of Health Sciences, College of Podiatric Medicine, Pomona,
California, USA

ROBERT D. PHILLIPS, DPM
Orlando VA Medical Center, Program Director, Podiatric Medicine and Surgery
Residency, Professor, Podiatric Medicine, University of Central Florida College of
Medicine, Orlando, Florida, USA

DOUGLAS RICHIE, DPM, FACFAS
Associate Clinics Professor, Applied Biomechanics, California School of Podiatric
Medicine at Samuel Merritt University, Oakland, California, USA

HAROLD D. SCHOENHAUS, DPM, FACFAS
Surgical Editor to Present E-learning, Attending Podiatric Physician, Penn Presbyterian
Medical Center, Professor, Temple University School of Podiatric Medicine, Philadelphia,
Pennsylvania, USA

JARROD SHAPIRO, DPM, FACFAS, FACFAOM
Associate Professor, Western University of Health Sciences, College of Podiatric
Medicine, Department of Podiatric Medicine, Surgery and Biomechanics, Program
Director, Chino Valley Medical Center Podiatric Medicine and Surgery Residency with
Rearfoot Reconstruction and Ankle Certificate, Pomona, California, USA

SCOTT SPENCER, DPM, FACFAOM
Associate Professor, Department of Surgery/Biomechanics, Kent State University College of Podiatric Medicine, Independence, Ohio, USA

JOHN TASSONE, DPM, FACFAOM
Associate Professor, Arizona School of Podiatric Medicine, Private Practice, Summit Medical Group, Glendale, Arizona, USA

AUDRIS TIEN, DPM
PGY-3, Podiatry Resident, 3rd Year, Podiatric Medicine and Surgery with Rearfoot Reconstruction and Ankle Certificate, Chino Valley Medical Center, Chino, California, USA

MELANIE VIOLAND, DPM, FACFAS
Associate Professor, Arizona School of Podiatric Medicine, Midwestern University, Glendale, Arizona, USA

Contents

In trying to explain the myriad of foot deformities and symptoms that have slow onset and/or are considered to be overuse syndromes, clinicians have been trying to develop quantitative examinations to describe the cause of the patient's problems and to better individualize treatment modalities. This type of examination is called a biomechanical examination. This article discusses some of the more common portions of a biomechanical examination of the foot and lower extremity. It will also point out some ways that the information from a biomechanical examination can be applied in clinically treating patients.

Imaging with biomechanical analysis augments the clinical examination and improves outcomes by correlating imaging findings with the examination. Plain film radiographs are the gold standard to assess osseous alignment. The biomechanical examination provides information to formulate an accurate assessment. Weightbearing computed tomography scanning is a potentially valuable for functional information about joint biomechanics. True alignment of the lower extremity can be appreciated on weightbearing computed tomography scanning. Soft tissue structures can be assessed with diagnostic ultrasound examination. Acute and chronic injuries that compromise joint stability can be identified.

Understanding of medial column biomechanics is paramount to a successful outcome in both conservative and surgical treatment. Dysfunctions of the dynamic stabilizers as well as the static stabilizers of the medial column play a role in pathomechanics. Conservative options for addressing the medial column include custom foot orthotics and bracing. Options for addressing the medial column surgically with the goal to restore a stable tripod configuration, include first tarsometatarsal joint arthrodesis, opening plantarflexory medial cuneiform osteotomy, and naviculocuneiform arthrodesis.

considerations. This article reviews the use of the 2 primary biomechanical approaches, the kinematic and kinetic methods, and presents a novel unified method to guide surgical procedure choice, the kineticokinematic approach. Decision-making methods and resources are discussed and 2 case studies are presented to elucidate how this method may be used when choosing surgical procedures.

This article discusses rearfoot fusions for foot and ankle surgeons. It establishes normal foot and ankle function primarily in the stance phase of gait. The foot is greatly affected by external and internal forces, which contribute to normal function or the need for compensatory mechanisms. As a result of compensation, many symptoms develop, often leading to debilitating disorders such as degenerative joint disease. The interaction of the ankle, subtalar, and midtarsal joints are outlined. Congenital deformities, trauma and abnormal compensation are reviewed along with corresponding sequelae. Surgery is often indicated to reduce symptoms, improve position, and help stabilize the foot.

The article discusses the nuances required to effectively perform the biomechanical examination in children and assess the findings. The author covers several factors in children that make the examination different in certain respects than in that of adults, including growth, osseous maturation, gait development, and interpretation of symptoms as conveyed by the child. Further delineation is made for prewalkers, foot-flat to foot-flat walkers, and heel-to-toe walkers. Segmental review of the lower extremity is covered by age bracket, with clinical pearls inserted where relevant to assist the clinician. A brief discussion of shoe wear and orthoses is made as well.

Biomechanical changes to the lower extremity in patients with diabetes mellitus are typically greatest with peripheral neuropathy, although peripheral arterial disease also impacts limb function. Changes to anatomic structures can impact daily function. These static changes, coupled with kinetic and kinematic changes of gait, lead to increased vertical and shear ground reactive forces, resulting in ulcerations. Unsteadiness secondary to diminished postural stability and increased sway increase fall risk. These clinical challenges and exacerbation of foot position and dynamic changes associated with limb salvage procedures, amputations, and prostheses are necessary and can impact daily function, independence, quality of life, and mortality.

A comprehensive lower extremity examination is a critical examination component for any type of injury in an athlete but should also be part of a preseason or preventive care program. Identification and treatment of biomechanical abnormalities and association with evidence-based risk factors for lower extremity disorders can be incorporated to potentially reduce risk or prevent acute and chronic injuries.

CLINICS IN PODIATRIC MEDICINE AND SURGERY

FORTHCOMING ISSUES

April 2020
Top Research in Podiatry Education
Thomas Chang, *Editor*

July 2020
OrthoplasticTechniques for Lower Extremity Reconstruction
Edgardo R. Rodriguez-Collazo and Suhail Masadeh, *Editors*

RECENT ISSUES

October 2019
Updates in Implants for Foot and Ankle Surgery: 35 Years of Clinical Perspectives
Meagan Jennings, *Editor*

July 2019
Diabetes
Paul Jeong Kim, *Editor*

SERIES OF RELATED INTEREST

Foot and Ankle Clinics
Available at: www.foot.theclinics.com
Orthopedic Clinics
Available at: www.orthopedic.theclinics.com

Foreword

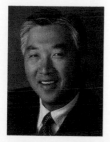

Thomas J. Chang, DPM
Consulting Editor

As I consider topics for the future issues of our *Clinics in Podiatric Medicine and Surgery*, it is clear that many of the prior issues have a surgical focus. It has been my hope to integrate more discussion on topics of Podiatric Medicine and nonsurgical areas of patient care. This issue is an attempt to offer more diversity, yet I realized early on that I have favored surgery once again. I learned within the first months of my tenure at the California College of Podiatric Medicine (CCPM) that surgery and biomechanics are intimately related. Many, if not all, of our surgical principles are based on the biomechanical principles and teachings. One simply cannot exist without the other, and there is no better area of the body where that holds true.

Much of the foot and ankle community is forever indebted to the early work done by Drs Root, Weed, and Orien. While at CCPM, I was grateful to Drs Jack Morris and Paul Scherer for their influence on many of our students and my career. There are so many names to recognize. Drs Richie, Kirby, Williams, and Huppin continue to challenge biomechanical principles in our current literature. Our international Podiatric colleagues, Drs Prior, Spooner, Payne, and Bartold, are well-respected leaders in this area and continue to educate on every continent.

As many of us aspire to be better foot and ankle surgeons, we should equally aspire to master biomechanics. Bone surgery is soundly rooted in structural and biomechanical principles. When we examine our surgical successes and failures, we are continuously reminded of whether or not we made sound biomechanical decisions.

I am grateful to Dr Shapiro and his efforts in creating this issue. I hope you enjoy this Biomechanics Update.

Thomas J. Chang, DPM
Redwood Orthopedic Surgery Associates
208 Concourse Boulevard
Santa Rosa, CA 95403, USA

E-mail address:
thomaschang14@comcast.net

Clin Podiatr Med Surg 37 (2020) xiii
https://doi.org/10.1016/j.cpm.2019.10.002
0891-8422/20/© 2019 Published by Elsevier Inc.

podiatric.theclinics.com

Preface

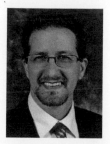

Jarrod Shapiro, DPM
Editor

This issue of *Clinics in Podiatric Medicine and Surgery* focuses on biomechanics of the foot and ankle. I have chosen to highlight the work of thought-leaders from around the United States to provide a broad evidence-based survey of various issues pertinent to lower-extremity biomechanics. The articles cover a range of subjects from principles of biomechanics (including examination fundamentals and discussions of the medial and lateral columns of the foot) to the use of imaging to surgical biomechanics and decision making. Specific subjects, such as diabetes, sports medicine, and podopediatrics, as well as the use of orthoses for adult-acquired flatfoot deformity, delve deeply into the specifics to provide useful information for practitioners. I hope this issue delivers a comprehensive review of an important core aspect of foot and ankle medicine and surgery.

Also, I want to dedicate this issue to the late Paul Scherer, DPM. Dr Scherer was a teacher, researcher, expert biomechanist, and universally respected leader in the profession. It is my hope that Dr Scherer would have enjoyed reading and discussing the varied topics in this issue. All of our best wishes go out to his family. Thank you for being a true mentor to a thankful profession.

Jarrod Shapiro, DPM
Western University of Health Sciences
College of Podiatric Medicine
Department of Podiatric Medicine, Surgery and Biomechanics
Chino Valley Medical Center Podiatric Medicine and
Surgery Residency with Rearfoot Reconstruction and Ankle Certificate
795 East 2nd Street, Suite 7
Pomona, CA 91766, USA

E-mail address:
Jarrod0517@gmail.com

Clin Podiatr Med Surg 37 (2020) xv
https://doi.org/10.1016/j.cpm.2019.10.001
0891-8422/20/© 2019 Published by Elsevier Inc.

Using the Biomechanical Examination to Guide Therapy

Robert D. Phillips, DPM[a,b,c,]*

KEYWORDS

- Biomechanics • Goniometry • Abnormal foot function

KEY POINTS

- Biomechanical examination is a general term to define an examination that defines whether abnormal mechanical function of a body part is occurring.
- The first goal of the biomechanical examination is to identify that abnormal function is occurring.
- The second goal of the biomechanical examination is to identify the cause of the abnormal function.
- The third goal of the biomechanical examination is to link the abnormal function with the reasons for the pathologic condition developing, or it should predict pathologic condition that is likely to develop.
- The biomechanical examination is a composite of evaluating function, joint range of motion, and testing for muscle tension and strength.

The biomechanical examination is much more complex than can be considered in a short article. In summary, it is an examination of the musculoskeletal system in a way that a predictive model can be assembled to identify why performance is suboptimal or symptomatic and how function can be modified and enhanced. It is usually the identification of variables that create normal and abnormal ambulatory activities, standing and walking being the most common.

The terms normal and abnormal are in themselves ambiguous terms and have been debated over the years. Two common uses relate back to the ideas of Aristotle and Plato. Those who follow the ideas of Plato relate normal as being the average, whereas those on the Aristotelian side think of normal as being ideal. Thus, when considering the literature on the subject of normal foot function, the reader has to first ask himself or herself whether the authors of the research believe in the Platonic or the Aristotelian

Disclosure Statement: The author has nothing to disclose.
[a] Orlando VA Medical Center, Orlando, FL, USA; [b] Podiatric Medicine and Surgery Residency;
[c] Podiatric Medicine, University of Central Florida College of Medicine, Orlando, FL, USA
* 13800 Veterans Way, Orlando, FL 32825.
E-mail addresses: Robert.Phillips9@va.gov; rdpvamc@gmail.com

line of thinking. Frederic Wood Jones (1875–1954) expressed the difficulty of accepting an Aristotelian attitude toward the foot with these words, "It is a little difficult to know why the human foot should be selected as an organ that is assumed to have an ideal or perfect form differing from that which the anatomist finds to be normal in the vast majority of mankind. If we substitute 'normal' for 'ideal' in the above sentence, we must conclude that the bulk of humanity is condemned by the normal disposition of the bones of the foot to show some departure from the normal functioning of the foot. The only alternative is to assume that there is such a thing as ideal foot function and that this function could be presumably carried out by an ideal but not by the normal foot."[1]

Merton L. Root defined a normal foot in these terms: ""The term normal represents a set of circumstances whereby the foot will function in a manner which will not create adverse physical or emotional response in the individual. This definition applies when the lower extremity is used in an average manner and in an average environment, as dictated by the needs of society at the moment."[2] Of course, this definition leaves many questions unanswered. What constitutes an adverse physical response? What constitutes an adverse emotional response? What is an average manner of use? What is an average environment? What are the needs of society?

These questions, then, show that the definition of normal shifts quickly and can vary from moment to moment. Is the ability to run more than 50 miles per week normal? If a person's foot can withstand the stresses of average activity without any adverse effect for 30 years, does that mean that same foot can withstand the stresses of average activity for another 30 years? Most research studies that have tried to define the characteristics of a normal foot have studied young people. The fallacy of this has been recognized, and now there are longitudinal studies to better find those characteristics of those feet that do not suffer adverse effects over many years.[3,4]

So what is a biomechanical examination? A biomechanical examination can be broken down into asking the following questions: (1) Is there abnormal function that is producing distress or producing inefficient performance? (2) Is there a cause of the abnormal function? (3) What is the cascade of events from the cause to the final function and symptoms? Any examination that answers any of these questions may be considered a biomechanical examination. Of course, the full biomechanical examination will answer all of these questions. Once one answers these questions, developing a strategy to correct the abnormal function becomes much easier.

First of all, is the identification of deviations of function from accepted standards of normal? It is not within the scope of this article to identify how these accepted standards are established. The 2 basic functions of the foot are standing and walking. Before walking, the standing evaluation is usually performed. Stance evaluation is often said to be done with the patient in their angle and base of gait. The angle of gait is usually assessed by watching the patient walk and then trying to reproduce that angle with the patient in static stance. The base of gait is considered the distance between the heels when viewed on the coronal plane in gait. Although there is some difference between the upper body position to the center of the foot during single support, there is a fairly good relationship between the maximum heel eversion in walking and the relaxed calcaneal stance position.[5]

The first static measurement that is helpful for making treatment decisions is the relaxed calcaneal stance position. It is commonly assumed that when the posterior calcaneal bisection is perpendicular to the ground, that an axial force from the leg downward is aligned with the center of pressure under the heel and the center of mass of the calcaneus and the talus. No one has proved this yet, but using the posterior calcaneal bisector as a prime marker assumes that it overlies the center of mass of the calcaneus. For reliability, it is recommended that the calcaneal bisection be made using a caliper.[6] It is also recommended that every time the foot moves to a different position that the calcaneus be rebisected because of skin movement over the os calcis.[7] Calculations predict minimum inversion, or eversion moments of the heel are achieved when the heel is vertical and centered under the leg. Therefore, it is commonly accepted that a major goal of therapy, whether it be conservative or surgical, is to bring the posterior calcaneal bisector into a vertical alignment with the ground so that a vertical line can be drawn through the center of the knee joint, center of the ankle joint, and center of the heel pad.[8]

How to identify excess rearfoot and midfoot pronation or supination in static stance has been greatly discussed in the literature for more than 100 years. There have been many measurements that have been proposed, some of them better validated and others more useful. The identification of a position of neutrality of the foot, mainly the subtalar joint, has been of great use, in describing foot function and is still a cornerstone of much therapy provided, although it continues to be highly debated.[9]

Before talking about any usefulness of a subtalar joint neutral position, it must be pointed out that to even state that the foot is in a pronated or supinated position, one has to have a reference position from which to measure. This reference position is usually called the neutral position. This is purely an existence statement and can neither be proved nor disproved by any scientific experiment.[10] Lovett and Cotton[11] identified a desired position of the foot with the words, "In contrast to the word pronation, the word supination will be used here to designate the corrected position of the foot in which, by the influence of voluntary muscular contraction, the foot is placed with its outer border touching the ground, in its normal relation to the leg, with the inner malleolus not unduly prominent." Creer[12] described the neutral position of the foot, in which the foot was balanced under the leg when there was an axial load and no muscle action. Wright and colleagues[13] described the neutral position as, "... the position of the ankle and subtalar joint when the subject was standing relaxed with the knees fully extended, the arms at the sides, feet six inches apart, and a comfortable amount of toeing-out." They then noted that during gait there was both eversion and inversion of the foot around this neutral position that has been accepted as being the normal motion. McPoil and Cornwall[14] also showed the same result and therefore proposed accepting the Wright and colleagues concept. There have been many other proposals for determining where the neutral position lies.

Although many use an alignment of the posterior heel and the posterior leg bisector as the definition of neutral,[15] Root[2] put forth several clinical identifying marks for determining neutral position. He considered that neutral was a point of posterior subtalar joint congruity on the medial and lateral sides. Others proposed that the congruity of joint surfaces is at the talonavicular joint.[16] Root also proposed a mathematical determination of neutral position, which was one-third of the way from the joint's fully pronated position and two-thirds of the way from the joint's fully supinated position. Phillips and Phillips[17] reported that the subtalar joint neutral position varied between individuals; however, the population average was very close to the ratio that Root proposed. This same variability and population average were supported with radiographic data from Bailey and colleagues.[18] The importance of this published data is that clinicians should review their range-of-motion results over a period of time, and although they may find that many of their patients do not have the one-third to two-third ratio of motion between pronation and supination from neutral, that their population average should be close to that. If it does not, the clinician needs to reevaluate their techniques of measurement.

This author has concluded the Root concept of neutral to be the most useful clinically. A major reason is that many individuals are noted to stand with the heel vertical or with the heel and leg in alignment, yet they exhibit signs and symptoms of excessive rearfoot pronation (**Fig. 1**). When one places the subtalar joint in a state of congruity, they often find that the heel is in an inverted or everted state relative to the ground or the leg. Root introduced the concept that certain people may have the heel inverted or everted from the leg when the subtalar joint is in neutral position, and although the heel may be in line with the leg in stance, the person may suffer from symptoms associated with excessive pronation or excessive supination. Only by knowing how the heel alignment to the leg compares in static stance with that when the subtalar joint is palpated to be in neutral position can one make any statement as to whether the person is standing with the subtalar joint pronated or supinated.[19] Houck and colleagues[20] demonstrated that graphing subtalar joint motion in gait relative to a Root-neutral position versus graphing motion relative to a vertical "neutral position" would describe motion that is more consistent with whether the person experiences symptoms consistent with abnormal pronation or supination.

There have been many proposed reasons a major objective of treatment, whether it be bracing, shoes, orthoses, exercise, or surgery, is to push the subtalar joint toward its neutral position in stance. Pushing the joint toward a position of greater joint congruity will theoretically spread out joint forces over a greater surface area and decrease the likelihood of osteoarthritis. It is hypothesized that when the subtalar joint is in neutral position there should be a balance between the passive tension in the invertor and evertor muscles of the rearfoot. When the subtalar joint pronates, the posterior tibial tendon is lengthened, which decreases its maximum contractile force and could lead to posterior tibial tendinitis and possibly posterior tibial tendon failure.[21] Likewise, when the subtalar joint supinates, the peroneus brevis is stretched, decreasing its maximum contraction force, which could lead to peroneal tendinitis.

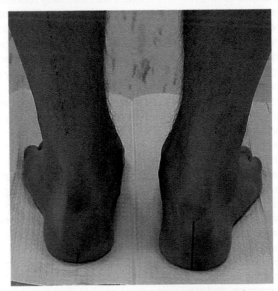

Fig. 1. Vertical calcaneus in stance, yet patient has very pronated foot as noted by the forefoot abduction and the prominence of the head of the talus on the medial side. This argues that vertical calcaneus does not mean that the subtalar joint is in its neutral position.

Considering the passive tension in the invertors and evertors of the foot is especially important in people with diseases that affect the integrity of the soft tissues. Rheumatoid arthritis is one particular disease that weakens all of the collagen tissues, including all tendons; thus, posterior tibial dysfunction is a higher risk in these patients.[22] Therefore, it can be argued that clinicians should be much more aggressive in prophylactically treating patients with rheumatoid arthritis, especially if the foot is already highly pronated.[23,24]

When one knows how much the subtalar joint is abnormally pronating, then a better estimate can be made as to the aggressiveness of the therapy. There are certain causes of pronation that may not be amenable to orthotic therapy. Moderate to severe posterior tibial dysfunction will produce a degree of subtalar joint pronation that may need ankle-foot orthosis (AFO) bracing or even surgery rather than orthotics. A medially displaced subtalar joint axis may require modifications to orthotics to increase supination torques around the subtalar joint axis. One modification that has been proposed is to skive away some of the positive mold of the foot under the medial heel.[25] Another similar effect can be accomplished by using the inverted cast technique proposed for runners by Ferguson and Blake.[26] Certainly, this second technique has been shown to markedly decrease the force that is provided by the posterior tibial muscle to slow pronation as the foot hits the ground.[27] People with symptoms, in whom the subtalar joint is not maximally pronated, may be very adequately accommodated with orthoses that are preformed.

For those patients who have a high degree of subtalar joint pronation, yet the calcaneus is vertical or even inverted in static stance, trying to bring the calcaneus to vertical may not be adequate to alleviate symptoms. The term "partially compensated rearfoot varus" refers to that foot in which the subtalar joint is maximally pronated but the heel is inverted relative to the ground in static stance. Many inexperienced clinicians will confuse an inverted calcaneus in static stance as always being a supinated foot.[28,29] Without a knowledge of where the pronation end range of motion (EROM) of the subtalar joint lies, the clinician does not know for sure that observed inverted calcaneus in stance is really a pronated, neutral, or supinated foot. By performing a range-of-motion examination of the subtalar joint, the confusion as to whether this person standing with an inverted calcaneus is standing with the subtalar joint supinated or pronated is eliminated. For those patients standing with the subtalar joint supinated and the calcaneus inverted, the clinician will use therapy that will move the calcaneus toward the vertical position. In those patients standing with the subtalar joint pronated and the calcaneus inverted, the clinician will need to move the calcaneus into even a more inverted position, a little less pronated. For those patients with a partially compensated rearfoot varus, it is a mistake to make an AFO that would try to bring the heel vertical to the ground.

Identification of an abnormal subtalar joint axis is a very important part of the biomechanical examination. Phillips and Lidtke[30,31] used in vivo measurements to support the Kirby proposition that the subtalar joint axis projection onto the plantar foot should lie between the first and second metatarsal heads when the subtalar joint is in its neutral position. When it is in this position, normal ground forces produce an equilibrium of inversion-eversion torques around the subtalar joint axis. Pronation of the subtalar joint moves the axis medially, which increases pronation torque from vertical ground forces. In contrast, supination of the subtalar joint moves the axis laterally, which increases supination torque from vertical ground forces (**Fig. 2**).

When the subtalar joint axis is too far medial, standard orthotic therapy may not be enough to give adequate relief of symptoms (**Fig. 3**). In some people, surgery may be the best option. Phillips[32] proposed 2 types of medially displaced subtalar joint axes.

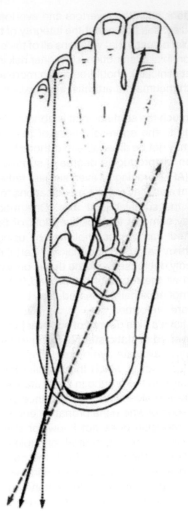

Fig. 2. The relationship of the subtalar joint axis with the plantar foot. The black arrow shows when the subtalar joint is in its neutral position; the blue arrow shows when the subtalar joint is maximally supinated, and the red arrow shows when the subtalar joint is in its fully pronated position. Once the foot pronates to the point that the subtalar joint moves medial to the first metatarsal head, it will then pronate to its end range of motion. For this reason, the degree of pronation may not be highly related to the degree of primary. For this reason, the degree of pronation may not be highly related to the degree of primary varus in the forefoot. The higher the amount of transverse plane dominance in the subtalar and midtarsal joint, the greater the medial movement of the subtalar joint axis when the rearfoot pronates. (*From* Phillips, Robert D., and Roy H. Lidtke. "Clinical determination of the linear equation for the subtalar joint axis." Journal of the American Podiatric Medical Association 82, no. 1 (1992): 1-20; with permission.)

Type I shows the axis normally located under the heel, but has a high angle to the sagittal plane so that it is medial to the first metatarsal head. The Evans osteotomy, which lengthens the lateral column, may be the choice because it has the effect of moving the forefoot medial to the subtalar joint axis.[33] Type II shows the axis located

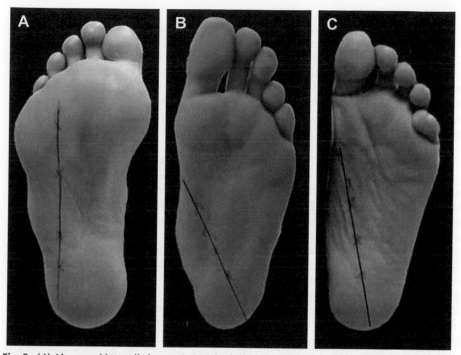

Fig. 3. (*A*) Abnormal laterally located subtalar joint axis. This type of foot is highly supinated in stance. Treatment must concentrate on increasing the force or lever arm lateral to the axis. (*B*) Abnormal type I medially located subtalar joint axis. (*C*) Abnormal type II medially located subtalar joint axis. Both types of medially located subtalar joint axis require treatments that increase ground reaction force medial to the axis; however, there may be differences in both conservative and surgical treatment. Type I is more likely to respond to techniques to increase force under the medial heel pad than type II. Surgery for type I needs a procedure to only move the forefoot medial to the axis, whereas type II needs a procedure to also move the rearfoot medial to the axis.

too far medial under the heel and under the forefoot. With this type of foot, surgery such as a calcaneal osteotomy to move the heel medially may be necessary.[34]

When the subtalar joint is in neutral position, the midtarsal joint has a smaller range of motion than when the subtalar joint is pronated. As the subtalar joint supinates when weightbearing, the forefoot has to pronate, which decreases tension in the plantar fascia and allows the metatarsophalangeal joints to dorsiflex.[35] Finally, supination of the subtalar joint is necessary during the propulsive period of gait, which allows the first metatarsal to plantarflex relative to the rearfoot, which, with the decrease in tension in the plantar fascia, creates first metatarsophalangeal joint dorsiflexion, heel lift, ankle joint plantarflexion, knee flexion, and hip extension. The combined actions in these joints increase stride length and also improves the lordotic curve of the lumbar spine.[36]

The forefoot-to-rearfoot relationship has always been considered an important part of any biomechanical assessment. It has been long recognized that the forefoot needs to contact the ground, and that the foot will do what is necessary to try to bring all 5 metatarsal heads to the ground during midstance. Of particular importance is assessing whether the first metatarsal head can touch the ground (**Fig. 4**).[37,38] If it cannot, then the usual action is pronation of the rearfoot and midfoot so that the first metatarsal head can touch the ground.[39] On the other hand, a person with a forefoot valgus can stand with the subtalar joint in neutral position, and a valgus wedge can be inserted under the forefoot with no discomfort to the patient and no change in the heel-to-ground relationship (**Fig. 5**). It has been demonstrated that there is a relationship between the presence of forefoot varus and pronation of the subtalar joint in static stance so that the first metatarsal touch will be the ground. However, in mild cases of forefoot varus, the calcaneus may evert more than the degree of forefoot varus measured.[40] This greater pronation than would be predicted by the amount of forefoot varus is because as the subtalar joint pronates, the axis moves medial to the first metatarsal head, and that movement may be to the point that the subtalar joint will be forced to pronate to its end range of motion.

Many methodologies have been proposed for assessing the forefoot-to-rearfoot relationship.[41,42] Root and colleagues stated that the assessment should be made when the subtalar joint is neutral and the midtarsal joint is fully pronated. In doing so, they had accepted the Elftman hypothesis for the pronation end range of motion of the midtarsal joint.[43] However, after proving that the end range of motion is not an osseous locking mechanism, it became clear that the amount of force used to pronate the midtarsal joint determined the angle between the forefoot and the rearfoot.[44] Unfortunately, no study has been published that relates the angle of the forefoot to rearfoot with the amount of force used to pronate the midtarsal joint. With no such standardization, it is little wonder that there have been such wide variations in the intratester and intertester reliability to measure such an angle.[45,46] As this author has analyzed the clinical technique of Root from personal observation, he has concluded that the Root technique finds the forefoot maximally pronated position at that position from which further pronation force against the forefoot produces a subtalar joint pronation from its neutral position.

The controversies about the value of the forefoot-to-rearfoot relationship may be more due to the fact that evaluation of the forefoot-to-rearfoot relationship using a single measurement may not be adequate for fully assessing the function of the foot.[47] It has long been recognized that there is a twisting action of the forefoot against the

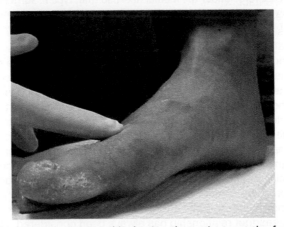

Fig. 4. True forefoot varus is diagnosed by having the patient rest the foot on the ground with the subtalar joint in neutral position. Pressure downward on the first metatarsal head will not be able to push the first metatarsal down to the ground. An orthosis must support the forefoot inverted relative to the ground. An accurate measure of how much wedging is desirable is part of the biomechanical examination. A wedge only under the forefoot with no supination force under the heel will cause the forefoot to invert more, and the patient will pronate off the forefoot wedge.

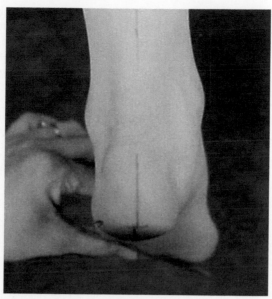

Fig. 5. Forefoot valgus diagnosed by noting the forefoot is everted to the calcaneal bisection when the subtalar joint is in neutral position and the forefoot is fully pronated against the rearfoot. This can be confirmed by placing a wedge under the lateral column of the forefoot when the patient is standing in neutral position and noting no pronation of the subtalar joint. The clinician will find that the patient is much more stable in the ankle as well as their general posture when such forefoot valgus wedge is built into an insole of the shoe.

rearfoot during any plantigrade function of the foot.[48,49] Because the 5 metatarsal heads maintain contact with the ground during midstance, if the rearfoot everts from being perpendicular, the forefoot has to invert relative to the rearfoot in order for the 5 metatarsal heads to stay in contact with the ground (**Fig. 6**). Where this motion occurs in the midfoot may vary from person to person.[50] In some individuals, the motion may occur as a true frontal plane motion in the midtarsal joint. In other individuals, there may be sagittal plane motions in any of the lesser tarsal joints or the metatarsotarsal joints. For example, the medial cuneiform may dorsiflex, to create an inverted forefoot to rearfoot position, which would cause the heel to evert in stance. The stiffness of these various joints in the midfoot will determine how much the heel can evert in stance.[51] It will also determine the stress and strain in and around the joints of the foot. As an example, this author has observed clinically a tendency for patients who have hallux valgus to have less frontal plane mobility of the midtarsal joint and a higher amount of mobility in the first metatarsocuneiform and cuneiform-navicular joints. New kinematic data in young pain-free individuals point to as much motion occurring in the tarsometatarsal and lesser tarsal joints as in the midtarsal joint during gait.[52] How the actual kinematic motions of all these joints relate to the range of motion available in these small forefoot joints is still unknown and needs more research.

Using the concept of the forefoot twisting in the opposite direction to the rearfoot when one is standing, it can be seen that if the clinician prevents the forefoot from inverting to the rearfoot, then the patient will be unable to evert the calcaneus from perpendicular when standing. Likewise, if the clinician blocks the forefoot from everting to the rearfoot, the patient will be unable to invert the heel from perpendicular when

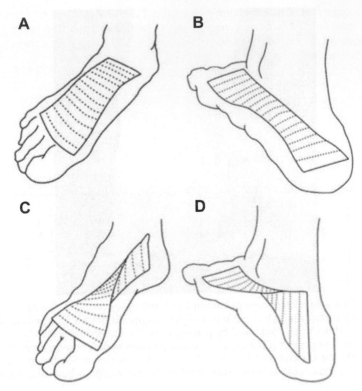

Fig. 6. The twisted plate concept was proposed by MacConnaill. (*A, B*) As the heel everts in static stance, the forefoot has to invert to the rearfoot. This increases the tension in the plantar fascia. (*C, D*) As the heel inverts in static stance, the forefoot everts to the rearfoot. This decreases the tension in the plantar fascia. If the forefoot is blocked from inverting to the rearfoot in static stance, the heel cannot evert from being perpendicular. Root orthotic theory is built on this concept as are many of the surgeries for flat foot. (*Reprinted from Journal of Biomechanics, Vol 93, Issue 93, Araújo VL, Souza TR, Magalhães FA, et al. Effects of a foot orthosis inspired by the concept of a twisted osteoligamentous plate on the kinematics of foot-ankle complex during walking: A proof of concept, Pages No., Copyright 2019, with permission from Elsevier.*)

standing. For this reason, Steindler[53] proposed that to correct a flat foot with shoe wedging, one needed not only a varus wedge under the heel but also a valgus wedge under the forefoot. Root and colleagues[54] developed their casting technique using a non-weight-bearing impression in which the subtalar joint was not just placed in its neutral position, but the forefoot was everted to its maximum point. By using a fairly rigid material, the Root orthosis is intended to provide a varus twisting action to the calcaneus, and also resist the varus twisting of the forefoot against the rearfoot during in stance. The greater the resistance to the forefoot varus twisting aginst the rearfoot, the more effective the Root orthotic will be. Trying to understand where the excess forefoot-to-rearfoot inversion occurs may also be very important to analyze when considering surgical correction of the flatfoot deformity. Various arthrodesis procedures have been developed on the medial column of the foot to prevent pronation that cannot be stopped with more conservative orthotic and bracing methodologies. Young's tenosuspension uses the anterior tibial tendon to reinforce the ligaments under the medial metatarsocuneiform joint and naviculocuneiform joint. This reinforce-ment can markedly reduce the inversion of the forefoot against the rearfoot if that inversion occurs at the medial lesser tarsal joints; however, it does nothing to stop inversion of the forefoot against the rearfoot at the midtarsal joint.[55]

The relationship between the mobility of the forefoot and the position of the subtalar joint was a focus of attention by Elftman and Manter.[56] They formulated a theory of calcaneocuboid and talonavicular joint axes intersecting to explain this relationship. The postulates of Root incorporated the mobility concept of Elftman, but are not totally dependent on the Elftman postulate. Phillips and Phillips attempted to measure the change in the forefoot-to-rearfoot relationship for various subtalar joint positions. They produced a graph of this relationship for the forefoot fully pronated position. **Fig. 7** is the average of all their subjects. Since the submission of this article, no addi-tional research has confirmed or refuted their findings. On the graph, the x-axis is the position of the subtalar joint, and the y-axis is the forefoot-to-rearfoot relationship. As noted, as the subtalar joint pronates, the forefoot becomes exponentially more everted to the rearfoot. To use this in a clinic situation, one compares this curve with the "y = −x" line, to find out how much the midfoot has to supinate on the frontal plane to compensate for each degree of subtalar joint pronation. For example, if the patient stands with the heel vertical, the forefoot hits the ground with the midfoot fully pronated. If the heel everts 4°, then the forefoot has to invert 7° from its fully pronated position. If the heel everts 10°, then the forefoot has to invert 21° from its fully pronated position. Of course, this graph is only an average, with great variations in the population.

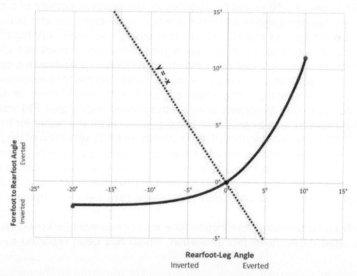

Fig. 7. The average forefoot-to-rearfoot relationship when forefoot is maximally pronated against the rearfoot, for various positions of the subtalar joint. The dotted line represents what happens in stance, meaning that the forefoot everted to the rearfoot when the rear-foot is inverted from perpendicular, and the forefoot is inverted to the rearfoot when the rearfoot is everted from perpendicular. If the forefoot is prevented from inverting to the rearfoot, the patient cannot evert the heel from being perpendicular to the ground. (*Data from* Phillips, R. D., and R. L. Phillips. "Quantitative analysis of the locking position of the midtarsal joint." Journal of the American Podiatry Association 73, no. 10 (1983): 518-522.)

The importance of this graph is to understand orthotic therapy. Most research on orthotic therapy has shown that although a foot is casted in neutral position, the orthotic may decrease the amount and velocity of pronation, yet it usually fails to bring the subtalar joint to neutral position.[57–59] This means that the orthotic has flexed from the shape that it was made to. Almost no research exists on how much orthotics flex when subjects stand on them. In some patients, when it is recognized that the subtalar joint is pronating when the patient stands on the orthotic, and it is not possible or not desirable to move the subtalar joint closer to its neutral position, the patient may continue to complain of pain under the medial side of the foot or the patient may feel unstable, like they are sliding laterally. These complaints can be solved by everting the forefoot closer to its fully pronated position. To do this, an extra wedge is added on top of the orthotic, under the forefoot (**Fig. 8**).

Some degree of midtarsal and forefoot joint function can be assessed using various foot posture indices. The Foot Posture Index (FPI) has become very popular in recent years. It is a quasiquantitative way of combining many of the signs of abnormal pronation or supination to categorize feet.[60] It is the summation of 6 different clinical signs that may be used to identify abnormal pronation of the subtalar joint and midtarsal joint. For each of these signs, a value of −2 to +2 is qualitatively assigned by the examiners and then added up for a final score. The 6 items are as follows: (1) palpation of the talar head in the navicular acetabulum, (2) congruity of the curvatures above and below the lateral malleolus, (3) the inverted or everted state of the calcaneus in static stance, (4) the medial bulge of the talonavicular joint, (5) the congruence of the medial longitudinal arch, and (6) the abduction or adduction of the forefoot against the rearfoot. A score of +16 would be possible for the greatest amount of pronation of both joints, and a score of −16 would be possible for the greatest amount of supination. A score of +4 has been shown to be the average in an asymptomatic population.[61] One of the advantages of the FPI is that its reliability has been very high.[62,63] The FPI does not identify causes of excessive pronation, and it does not divide the abnormal pronation into forefoot and rearfoot pronation or supination, except generally. The FPI has been shown to be very helpful in predicting risk for various pathologic conditions. Postural stability is decreased as the FPI increases.[64] Knee osteoarthritis and patellofemoral pain syndrome are also associated with higher FPI values.[65,66] Peak plantar pressure has been shown to be greater under the hallux for those with higher FPI.[67–69] Those with higher FPI also have higher EMG activation of the posterior tibialis and anterior tibialis muscles and lower peroneus longus activity.[70] The FPI has little use in defining the exact treatment needed; however, it is very valuable in identifying those individuals who are at greatest risk of developing problems and may be used as justification to instigate prophylactic treatment before symptoms manifest themselves.

Other indices for defining foot function have also been developed over the years. A commonly used measure of foot pronation, which has been reported to be fairly

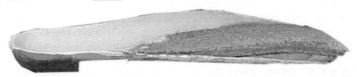

Fig. 8. Orthotic that cannot bring subtalar joint to neutral position but is modified by adding a valgus wedge under the forefoot to further pronate the forefoot closer to its end range of motion.

reliable, is the navicular drop.[71] The clinician finds a point on the medial navicular tuberosity and measures its height above the floor when the patient is sitting, foot on floor and the subtalar joint is in neutral position, and then again when the patient stands up. Average drop values of about 5 mm are considered normal; however, as the foot elongates, the normal navicular drop values are greater.[72] The navicular drop test is a direct measure of sagittal plane pronation of the midtarsal joint combined with dorsiflexion of the first ray. One may then infer an approximation of subtalar joint pronation; however, no studies have shown the relationship between these 2 variables. The weakness of the navicular drop is that it does not tell the practitioner whether the subtalar joint and midtarsal joint have used their entire reserve of pronation. It also does not identify the amount of transverse plane pronation occurring in the subtalar or midtarsal joint in stance.

The identification of the planar dominance as the subtalar joint pronates may be helpful in deciding treatment modalities[73] (**Fig. 9**). Pronation of the subtalar joint produces internal rotation of the leg as does pronation of the midtarsal joint. The total amount of internal rotation is a combination of the pronation in both of these joints.[74] The greater the ratio of the transverse to frontal plane motion in the subtalar/midtarsal joint complex, the more likely the subject will suffer symptoms in the leg rather than the foot.[75] Trying to determine how much of the transverse plane motion is due to actual subtalar joint motion and how much is due to purely midtarsal joint motion can be very difficult. Although goniometric methods of measuring the transverse and frontal plane motion components of the total range of motion have been described, no goniometric methods have been described for analyzing the transverse plane motion in the midtarsal joint, especially for various positions of the subtalar joint.[76] By analyzing the various components in the FPI, one may estimate some idea of the contribution of each joint.

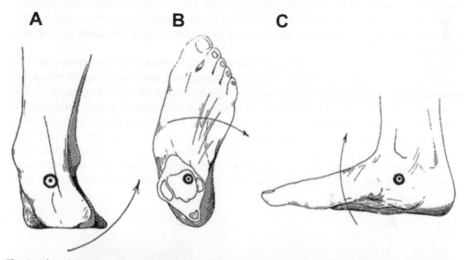

A   **B**   **C**

Fig. 9. Planal dominance of the subtalar and midtarsal joints will show different foot shapes in stance. (*A*) Frontal plane dominance will demonstrate a highly everted calcaneus, although the arch may not be highly collapsed. (*B*) Transverse plane dominance will show the forefoot more abducted against the rearfoot, giving the "too many toes" appearance. (*C*) Sagittal plane dominance will tend to show extremely low arch morphology with a pronated foot; however, very little forefoot abduction and very little calcaneus eversion may be noted. (*From* Green, D. R., and A. Carol. "Planal dominance." Journal of the American Podiatric Medical Association 74, no. 2 (1984): 98-103; with permission.)

However, when determining treatment, this division of transverse plane motion into the midtarsal and subtalar joints may make a difference in the treatment approach. If there is a high contribution by the midtarsal joint, then resistance to this pronation motion must occur more distally, not on the calcaneus. For orthotic therapy, this may require a high medial flange to prevent the medial movement of the talus.[77] On the other hand, if the planal dominance is more frontal in the subtalar joint, then long lever arms may be needed medially under the os calcis, such as flaring the orthotic heel posting more medially or even flaring the sole of the shoe medially (**Fig. 10**).

The effect of the length of the Achilles tendon needs to be considered when analyzing the cause of a pronated foot as well as the treatment needed. A short Achilles tendon has long been considered a cause of flat foot.[78–80] The ground reaction force under the metatarsal heads is proportional to the tension in the Achilles tendon.[81] This increase in ground reaction force under the forefoot produces an increase in the tension in the plantar fascia as well as the ligaments crossing the midtarsal joint.[82] At a certain point of tension in the plantar ligaments–which no one has actually determined, the midtarsal and subtalar joints pronate beyond the point of neutrality. The measurement of ankle joint dorsiflexion is usually done by placing 1 arm of a goniometer parallel to the long axis of the lower leg and the other arm of the goniometer parallel to the plantar surface of the foot. The examiner then places force against the forefoot to maximally dorsiflex the ankle joint while making sure not to allow the subtalar joint to pronate.[83,84] Unfortunately, every examiner will most likely place a different amount of force against the forefoot, which leads to intertester reliability variation (**Fig. 11**). It is most desirable to measure ankle joint dorsiflexion if one can control the torque being exerted around the ankle joint.[85,86] Some have postulated that the ankle joint dorsiflexion should be measured with the patient weight-bearing and leaning forward to determine the maximum dorsiflexion possible. This technique will almost always produce more dorsiflexion than a non-weight-bearing examination; however, the amount of torque around the ankle joint is also much greater.[87,88]

Most clinicians accept 10° of passive ankle joint dorsiflexion as being normal. This number is taken from the average maximum ankle joint dorsiflexion angle measured kinematically at the point of time when the heel is seen to lift from the ground.[89] Calculations also show that at about 10° of ankle joint dorsiflexion, which would be the point of heel lift, and the point at which the subtalar joint should be at its neutral position, the average moment around the ankle joint is between 0.4 and 0.5 Nm/kg.[90] Therefore, the ideal of measuring ankle joint dorsiflexion would be to take that measurement with the torque around the ankle joint standardized to the patient weight at that point when the heel is supposed to come off the ground. What may be even

A   **B**

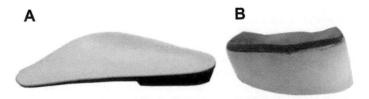

Fig. 10. (*A*) Orthotic has high medial flange to counter high transverse plane dominance in the subtalar and midtarsal joints abnormally pronating. (*B*) Orthotic has flare of the heel postmedially to increase supination moment arm of orthotic in a foot that has high frontal plane dominance. ([*A*] *Courtesy of* KLM Orthotic Laboratory, Valencia, CA; with permission.)

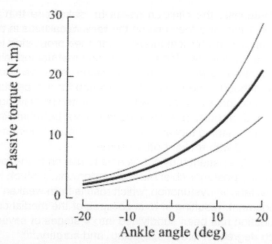

Fig. 11. As the Achilles tendon is stretched beyond its resting length, the passive tension starts producing plantarflexion torque around the ankle joint. This is considered the average torque for a normal population being produced around by this passive tension in the Achilles as the ankle joint is dorsiflexed. It is recommended that the clinician know about how much force he or she is placing against the forefoot when dorsiflexing the ankle joint, and then multiply that force by the distance from the ankle joint axis to the forefoot to calculate the torque being produced by the Achilles tendon. Much more research needs to be done to help clinicians decide when to diagnose a short Achilles tendon. (*From Moseley, Anne M., Jack Crosbie, and Roger Adams. "Normative data for passive ankle plantarflexion–dorsiflexion flexibility." Clinical Biomechanics 16, no. 6 (2001): 514-521; with permission.)*

more desirable is to produce the passive torque-angle curve over the entire ankle joint range of motion.[91,92] Some additional geometric calculations show that in stance, when the ankle joint is at 10° dorsiflexion, the center of body mass is over the first metatarsophalangeal joint. When the center of body mass passes from posterior to anterior over the metatarsophalangeal joint, the moment created by body weight around the joint changes from a plantarflexion to a dorsiflexion moment. This means that tall people will need to dorsiflex the ankle less than 10° to move the center of body mass forward of the metatarsophalangeal joint. Carrying a heavy backpack will move the center of mass posteriorly, which means a person may have to dorsiflex the ankle more than 10° to move the center of mass in front of the metatarsophalangeal joint. The clinician must, therefore, not consider 10° ankle joint dorsiflexion necessarily to be the criteria to fully define the Achilles as being short.

Treatment of a short Achilles tendon is usually a conservative approach. It is important to remember that the tension in the Achilles tendon in gait is a combination of passive tension plus active contraction of the triceps surae. Most of the time, isolated Achilles tendon lengthening is not indicated. Stretching exercises are usually used. Eccentric stretching exercises have become increasingly popular because the stretching is more concentrated in the tendon, and better increases in ankle joint range of motion are reported.[93,94]

Muscle testing is an important part of any biomechanical examination. For most clinicians, determination of strength is usually a qualitative examination; however, hand-held dynamometers have proven to be fairly reliable in giving clinicians more ability to quantitate muscle strength.[95] The triceps surae is the most difficult muscle to test for normal strength, because of its being the strongest muscle in the lower leg.[96,97] If there is a question of weakness, the clinician needs to make sure that the patient can adequately stand on 1 foot and then rise on the toes. Weakness in the triceps surae needs to be addressed with physical therapy. Because propulsion is a combination of knee joint flexion, ankle joint plantarflexion, and first metatarsophalangeal joint dorsiflexion, a weak triceps surae will result in a stiff knee in gait and a failure to propel.[98] A commonly thought, although unproven, compensation for triceps surae weakness is to use the long digital flexors to assist, which can be noted by clawing of the toes during late midstance and propulsion. If the triceps cannot be rehabilitated, bracing to prevent the patient from leaning forward too much at the ankle joint may be indicated, which may be combined with rocker bottom shoes.

Another reason that the patient may not be able to rise on to the toes in single support is weakness of the posterior tibial muscle tendon unit.[99] Much has been written about posterior tibial tendon dysfunction, which results from weakening and then failure of the spring ligament, resulting in total collapse of the medial column. Posterior tibial tendon dysfunction has been subdivided into 4 stages of severity, with recommendations in each degree for orthotic, bracing, and surgery.[100]

Peroneus brevis and longus weakness must be identified during the biomechanical examination. Peroneus brevis weakness may be a cause or a result of an abnormally supinated foot during gait. Because the peroneus brevis muscle lifts the lateral side of the foot, transferring weight to the medial side, if it is weakened, the clinician needs to add additional support under the lateral column of the forefoot. A great many of these patients will have a plantarflexed first ray and have a pes cavus appearance of the foot when sitting. It is preferable to take impressions of the foot with the patient sitting and dorsiflex the lateral column of the foot to its end range of motion. The support can then be made to hold the lateral column of the forefoot off the ground. It is fully expected that unless the peroneus brevis is strengthened, with time the patient will continue to develop an increasingly everted forefoot deformity.

Assessment of the plantar intrinsic muscle strength is another important part of the biomechanical examination.[101] Traditionally, it has been accepted that for static standing the intrinsic muscles are quiescent.[102] However, the intrinsics can be very important in creating the stiffening of the forefoot that is needed for generating strong propulsive power.[103] They have also been shown to decrease foot pronation during the midstance phase of gait.[104–106] Judging the strength of the intrinsics is difficult and qualitative, with few tools available to quantitate strength.[107,108] Because abnormal pronation of the foot may be caused by so many variables, many of which cannot be fixed, nevertheless, strengthening the intrinsic muscles of the foot may be a good adjunct in helping the pronated symptomatic foot more toward an asymptomatic foot.[109]

In conclusion, only a small snapshot of what comprises a biomechanical examination has been granted attention in this article. There are many other aspects that could be discussed. Range-of-motion availability is one very important part of the examination because it defines constraints within which the clinician must work. It may define the cause of abnormal pronation or supination; however, there are many causes that the goniometric examination cannot define. Without knowing the range of joint motions, clinicians may find themselves trying to build a brace or orthotic that tries to push a joint beyond its limitations, which will likely result in clinical failure and patient dissatisfaction. Reliability of joint range-of-motion examinations has been and will continue to be problematic; however, improved instrumentation and better definitions of techniques will improve this. Failure to continue to work on improved reliability will only result in degradation of clinicians' ability to fully analyze the causes of patient symptoms and also in decreasing the sophistication and individualization of the therapy provided. As one becomes more adept and complete in performing biomechanical examinations, new therapies become apparent. Certainly not all degrees of abnormal pronation or supination during the gait cycle can be solved with conservative methods, and for certain causes, a surgical approach may be better. However, without a full knowledge of the abnormal pronation cause and confounding variables, it is extremely easy to pick a surgical procedure that will not provide the optimal results. Therefore, the biomechanical examination may be more important for those patients for whom surgical intervention is contemplated.

REFERENCES

1. Jones FW. Structure and function as seen in the foot. Baillière, Tindall and Cox; 1944.
2. Root ML, Orien WP, Weed JH, et al. Biomechanical examination of the foot, vol. 1. Los Angeles: Clinical Biomechanics Corp; 1971.
3. Hill CL, Gill TK, Menz HB, et al. Prevalence and correlates of foot pain in a population-based study: the North West Adelaide health study. J Foot Ankle Res 2008;1(1):2–9.
4. Menz HB, Dufour AB, Katz P, et al. Foot pain and pronated foot type are associated with self-reported mobility limitations in older adults: the Framingham foot study. Gerontology 2016;62(3):289–95.
5. Donatelli R, Wooden M, Ekedahl SR, et al. Relationship between static and dynamic foot postures in professional baseball players. J Orthop Sports Phys Ther 1999;29(6):316–25.
6. LaPointe SJ, Peebles C, Nakra A, et al. The reliability of clinical and caliper-based calcaneal bisection measurements. J Am Podiatr Med Assoc 2001; 91(3):121–6.
7. Maslen BA, Ackland TR. Radiographic study of skin displacement errors in the foot and ankle during standing. Clin Biomech 1994;9(5):291–6.
8. Tateuchi H, Wada O, Ichihashi N. Effects of calcaneal eversion on three-dimensional kinematics of the hip, pelvis and thorax in unilateral weight bearing. Hum Mov Sci 2011;30(3):566–73.
9. Harradine P, Gates L, Bowen C. If it doesn't work, why do we still do it? The continuing use of subtalar joint neutral theory in the face of overpowering critical research. J Orthop Sports Phys Ther 2018;48(3):130–2.
10. Root ML. Biomechanical examination of the foot. J Am Podiatry Assoc 1973; 63(1):28–9.
11. Lovett RW, Cotton FJ. Some practical points in the anatomy of the foot. Boston Med Surg J 1898;139(5):101–7.
12. Creer WS. Some foot faults related to form and function. Br J Ind Med 1944;1(1): 54–61.
13. Wright DG, Desai SM, Henderson WH. Action of the subtalar and ankle-joint complex during the stance phase of walking. J Bone Joint Surg Am 1964; 46(2):361–464.
14. McPoil T, Cornwall MW. Relationship between neutral subtalar joint position and pattern of rearfoot motion during walking. Foot Ankle Int 1994;15(3):141–5.
15. American Academy of Orthopaedic Surgeons. Joint motion: method of measuring and recording. Chicago: Churchill Livingstone; 1965.
16. Wernick J, Langer S. A practical manual for a basic approach to biomechanics. New York: Langer Acrylic Laboratory; 1972.

17. Phillips RD, Phillips RL. Quantitative analysis of the locking position of the midtarsal joint. J Am Podiatry Assoc 1983;73(10):518–22.
18. Bailey DS, Perillo JT, Forman M. Subtalar joint neutral. A study using tomography. J Am Podiatr Med Assoc 1984;74(2):59–64.
19. Root ML. An approach to foot orthopedics. J Am Podiatry Assoc 1964;54(2): 115–8.
20. Houck JR, Tome JM, Nawoczenski DA. Subtalar neutral position as an offset for a kinematic model of the foot during walking. Gait Posture 2008;28(1):29–37.
21. Yeap JS, Singh D, Birch R. Tibialis posterior tendon dysfunction: a primary of secondary problem? Foot Ankle Int 2001;22(1):51–5.
22. Barn R, Turner DE, Rafferty D, et al. Tibialis posterior tenosynovitis and associated pes plano valgus in rheumatoid arthritis: electromyography, multisegment foot kinematics, and ultrasound features. Arthritis Care Res 2013;65(4):495–502.
23. Woodburn J, Barker S, Helliwell PS. A randomized controlled trial of foot orthoses in rheumatoid arthritis. J Rheumatol 2002;29(7):1377–83.
24. de P. Magalhaes E, Davitt M, Filho DJ, et al. The effect of foot orthoses in rheumatoid arthritis. Rheumatology 2005;45(4):449–53.
25. Bonanno DR, Zhang CY, Farrugia RC, et al. The effect of different depths of medial heel skive on plantar pressures. J Foot Ankle Res 2012;5(1):20–9.
26. Ferguson H, Blake RL. Update and rationale for the inverted functional foot orthosis. Clin Podiatr Med Surg 1994;11(2):311–37.
27. Baitch SP, Blake RL, Fineagan PL, et al. Biomechanical analysis of running with 25 degrees inverted orthotic devices. J Am Podiatr Med Assoc 1991;81(12): 647–52.
28. Tiberio D. Pathomechanics of structural foot deformities. Phys Ther 1988;68(12): 1840–9.
29. Vařeka I, Vařeková R. The height of the longitudinal foot arch assessed by Chippaux-Šmiřák index in the compensated and uncompensated foot types according to Root. Acta Univ Palacki Olomuc Gymn 2008;38(1):35–41.
30. Kirby KA. Methods for determination of positional variations in the subtalar joint Axis. J Am Podiatr Med Assoc 1987;77(5):228–34.
31. Phillips RD, Lidtke RH. Clinical determination of the linear equation for the subtalar joint axis. J Am Podiatr Med Assoc 1992;82(1):1–20.
32. Phillips RD. Chapter 5. Root theory: its origins and contemporary views. In: Albert SF, Curran SA, editors. Lower extremity biomechanics, theory and practice. Volume 1. Denver (CO): Bipedmed, LLC; 2013. p. 147–204.
33. Benthien RA, Parks BG, Guyton GP, et al. Lateral column calcaneal lengthening, flexor digitorum longus transfer, and opening wedge medial cuneiform osteotomy for flexible flatfoot: a biomechanical study. Foot Ankle Int 2007;28(1):70–7.
34. Kim JR, Shin SJ, Wang S-I, et al. Comparison of lateral opening wedge calcaneal osteotomy and medial calcaneal sliding-opening wedge cuboid-closing wedge cuneiform osteotomy for correction of planovalgus foot deformity in children. J Foot Ankle Surg 2013;52(2):162–6.
35. Sarrafian SK. Functional characteristics of the foot and plantar aponeurosis under tibiotalar loading. Foot Ankle 1987;8(1):4–18.
36. Dananberg HJ. Functional hallux limitus and its relationship to gait efficiency. J Am Podiatr Med Assoc 1986;76(11):648–52.
37. Morton DJ. Metatarsus atavicus: the identification of a distinctive type of foot disorder. J Bone Joint Surg 1927;9(3):531–44.
38. Perkins G. Pes planus or instability of the longitudinal arch: president's address. Proc R Soc Med 1948;41:31–40.

39. Karthikeyan G, Jayraj SJ, Narayanan V. Effect of forefoot type on postural stability–a cross sectional comparative study. Int J Sports Phys Ther 2015; 10(2):213–24.

40. Buchanan KR, Davis I. The relationship between forefoot, midfoot, and rearfoot static alignment in pain-free individuals. J Orthop Sports Phys Ther 2005;35(9): 559–66.

41. Garbalosa JC, McClure MH, Catlin PA, et al. The frontal plane relationship of the forefoot to the rearfoot in an asymptomatic population. J Orthop Sports Phys Ther 1994;20(4):200–6.

42. Jarvis HL, Nester CJ, Jones RK, et al. Inter-assessor reliability of practice based biomechanical assessment of the foot and ankle. J Foot Ankle Res 2012;5(1):14.

43. Elftman H. The transverse tarsal joint and its control. Clin Orthop Relat Res 1960; 16:41–6.

44. Blackwood CB, Yuen TJ, Sangeorzan BJ, et al. The midtarsal joint locking mechanism. Foot Ankle Int 2005;26(12):1074–80.

45. Somers DL, Hanson JA, Kedzierski CM, et al. The influence of experience on the reliability of goniometric and visual measurement of forefoot position. J Orthop Sports Phys Ther 1997;25(3):192–202.

46. Van Gheluwe B, Kirby KA, Roosen P, et al. Reliability and accuracy of biomechanical measurements of the lower extremities. J Am Podiatr Med Assoc 2002;92(6):317–26.

47. Buldt AK, Murley GS, Levinger P, et al. Are clinical measures of foot posture and mobility associated with foot kinematics when walking? J Foot Ankle Res 2015; 8(1):63–74.

48. MacConaill MA. The postural mechanism of the human foot. Proc R Ir Acad B 1944/1945;50:265–78.

49. Hicks JH. The mechanics of the foot. I. The joints. J Anat 1953;88:345–57.

50. Leardini A, Benedetti MG, Berti L, et al. Rear-foot, mid-foot and fore-foot motion during the stance phase of gait. Gait Posture 2007;25(3):453–62.

51. Allen MK, Cuddeford TJ, Glasoe WM, et al. Relationship between static mobility of the first ray and first ray, midfoot, and hindfoot motion during gait. Foot Ankle Int 2004;25(6):391–6.

52. Nester CJ, Jarvis HL, Jones RK, et al. Movement of the human foot in 100 pain free individuals aged 18–45: implications for understanding normal foot function. J Foot Ankle Res 2014;7(1):51–60.

53. Steindler A. The supinatory, compensatory torsion of the fore-foot in pes valgus. J Bone Joint Surg 1929;11(2):272–6.

54. Root ML, Weed JH, Orien WP. Neutral position casting techniques. Los Angeles: Clinical Biomechanics Corporation; 1971.

55. Dragonetti L, Ingraffia C, Stellari F. The Young tenosuspension in the treatment of abnormal pronation of the foot. J Foot Ankle Surg 1997;36(6):409–13.

56. Elftman H, Manter J. The evolution of the human foot, with especial reference to the joints. J Anat 1935;70(Pt 1):56–67.

57. Novick A, Kelley DL. Case study: position and movement changes of the foot with orthotic intervention during the loading response of gait. J Orthop Sports Phys Ther 1990;11(7):301–12.

58. Zifchock RA, Davis I. A comparison of semi-custom and custom foot orthotic devices in high- and low-arched individuals during walking. Clin Biomech 2008; 23(10):1287–93.

59. Maharaj JN, Cresswell AG, Lichtwark GA. The immediate effect of foot orthoses on subtalar joint mechanics and energetics. Med Sci Sports Exerc 2018;50(7): 1449–56.
60. Redmond AC, Crosbie J, Ouvrier RA. Development and validation of a novel rating system for scoring standing foot posture: the Foot Posture Index. Clin Biomech 2006;21(1):89–98.
61. Redmond AC, Crane YZ, Menz HB. Normative values for the foot posture index. J Foot Ankle Res 2008;1(1):6–15.
62. Morrison SC, Ferrari J. Inter-rater reliability of the Foot Posture Index (FPI-6) in the assessment of the paediatric foot. J Foot Ankle Res 2009;2(1):26–30.
63. Evans AM, Copper AW, Scharfbillig RW, et al. Reliability of the Foot Posture Index and traditional measures of foot position. J Am Podiatr Med Assoc 2003; 93(3):203–13.
64. Angin S, İlçin N, Yesilyaprak SS, et al. Prediction of postural sway velocity by Foot Posture Index, foot size and plantar pressure values in unilateral stance. Eklem Hastalik Cerrahisi 2013;24(3):144–8.
65. Levinger P, Menz HB, Fotoohabadi MR, et al. Foot posture in people with medial compartment knee osteoarthritis. J Foot Ankle Res 2010;3(1):29–36.
66. Neal BS, Griffiths IB, Dowling GJ, et al. Foot posture as a risk factor for lower limb overuse injury: a systematic review and meta-analysis. J Foot Ankle Res 2014;7(1):55–67.
67. Jonely H, Brismée J-M, Sizer PS Jr, et al. Relationships between clinical measures of static foot posture and plantar pressure during static standing and walking. Clin Biomech 2011;26(8):873–9.
68. Sánchez-Rodríguez R, Martínez-Nova A, Escamilla-Martínez E, et al. Can the Foot Posture Index or their individual criteria predict dynamic plantar pressures? Gait Posture 2012;36(3):591–5.
69. Lee JS, Kim KB, Jeong JO, et al. Correlation of foot posture index with plantar pressure and radiographic measurements in pediatric flatfoot. Ann Rehabil Med 2015;39(1):10.
70. Murley GS, Menz HB, Landorf KB. Foot posture influences the electromyographic activity of selected lower limb muscles during gait. J Foot Ankle Res 2009;2(1):35–43.
71. Picciano AM, Rowlands MS, Worrell T. Reliability of open and closed kinetic chain subtalar joint neutral positions and navicular drop test. J Orthop Sports Phys Ther 1993;18(4):553–8.
72. Nielsen RG, Rathleff MS, Simonsen OH, et al. Determination of normal values for navicular drop during walking: a new model correcting for foot length and gender. J Foot Ankle Res 2009;2(1):12–23.
73. Green DR, Carol A. Planal dominance. J Am Podiatr Med Assoc 1984;74(2): 98–103.
74. Nester CJ. Rearfoot complex: a review of its interdependent components, axis orientation and functional model. The Foot 1997;7(2):86–96.
75. Pierrynowski MR, Finstad E, Kemecsey M, et al. Relationship between the subtalar joint inclination angle and the location of lower-extremity injuries. J Am Podiatr Med Assoc 2003;93(6):481–4.
76. Phillips RD, Christeck R, Phillips RL. Clinical measurement of the axis of the subtalar joint. J Am Podiatr Med Assoc 1985;75(3):119–31.
77. Banwell HA, Mackintosh S, Thewlis D, et al. Consensus-based recommendations of Australian podiatrists for the prescription of foot orthoses for symptomatic flexible pes planus in adults. J Foot Ankle Res 2014;7(1):49–61.

78. Geist ES. The role of the tendo Achillis in the etiology of weak-foot. J Am Med Assoc 1913;61(23):2029–31.
79. Harris RI, Beath T. Hypermobile flat-foot with short tendo Achillis. J Bone Joint Surg Am 1948;30(1):116–50.
80. Kaufman KR, Brodine SK, Shaffer RA, et al. The effect of foot structure and range of motion on musculoskeletal overuse injuries. Am J Sports Med 1999; 27(5):585–93.
81. Aronow MS, Diaz-Doran V, Sullivan RJ, et al. The effect of triceps surae contracture force on plantar foot pressure distribution. Foot Ankle Int 2006;27(1):43–52.
82. Bolívar YA, Munuera PV, Padillo JP. Relationship between tightness of the posterior muscles of the lower limb and plantar fasciitis. Foot Ankle Int 2013; 34(1):42–8.
83. Tiberio D, Bohannon RW, Zito MA. Effect of subtalar joint position on the measurement of maximum ankle dorsiflexic. Clin Biomech 1989;4(3):189–91.
84. Gatt A, Chockalingam N, Chevalier TL. Sagittal plane kinematics of the foot during passive ankle dorsiflexion. Prosthet Orthot Int 2011;35(4):425–31.
85. Assal M, Shofer JB, Rohr E, et al. Assessment of an electronic goniometer designed to measure equinus contracture. J Rehabil Res Dev 2003;40(3):235–9.
86. Wilken J, Rao S, Estin M, et al. A new device for assessing ankle dorsiflexion motion: reliability and validity. J Orthop Sports Phys Ther 2011;41(4):274–80.
87. Bennell KL, Talbot RC, Wajswelner H, et al. Intra-rater and inter-rater reliability of a weight-bearing lunge measure of ankle dorsiflexion. Aust J Physiother 1998; 44(3):175–80.
88. Munteanu SE, Strawhorn AB, Landorf KB, et al. A weightbearing technique for the measurement of ankle joint dorsiflexion with the knee extended is reliable. J Sci Med Sport 2009;12(1):54–9.
89. Scott SH, Winter DA. Talocrural and talocalcaneal joint kinematics and kinetics during the stance phase of walking. J Biomech 1991;24(8):743–52.
90. Kuster M, Sakurai S, Wood GA. Kinematic and kinetic comparison of downhill and level walking. Clin Biomech 1995;10(2):79–84.
91. Chesworth BM. Reliability of a torque motor system for measurement of passive ankle joint stiffness in control subjects. Physiother Can 1988;40(5):300–3.
92. Moseley AM, Crosbie J, Adams R. Normative data for passive ankle plantarflexion–dorsiflexion flexibility. Clin Biomech (Bristol, Avon) 2001;16(6): 514–21.
93. Mahieu NN, McNair P, Cools ANN, et al. Effect of eccentric training on the plantar flexor muscle-tendon tissue properties. Med Sci Sports Exerc 2008; 40(1):117–23.
94. O'Sullivan K, McAuliffe S, DeBurca N. The effects of eccentric training on lower limb flexibility: a systematic review. Br J Sports Med 2012;46(12):838–45.
95. Mentiplay BF, Perraton LG, Bower KJ, et al. Assessment of lower limb muscle strength and power using hand-held and fixed dynamometry: a reliability and validity study. PLoS One 2015;10(10):e0140822.
96. Davis PR, McKay MJ, Baldwin JN, et al. Repeatability, consistency, and accuracy of hand-held dynamometry with and without fixation for measuring ankle plantarflexion strength in healthy adolescents and adults. Muscle Nerve 2017; 56(5):896–900.
97. Ancillao A, Palermo E, Rossi S. Validation of ankle strength measurements by means of a hand-held dynamometer in adult healthy subjects. J Sensors 2017;2017:1–8.

98. Apti A, Akalan NE, Kuchimov S, et al. Plantar flexor muscle weakness may cause stiff-knee gait. Gait Posture 2016;46:201–7.
99. Richie Jr, Douglas H. Biomechanics and clinical analysis of the adult acquired flatfoot. Clin Podiatr Med Surg 2007;24(4):617–44.
100. Pomeroy GC, Howard Pike R, Beals TC, et al. Acquired flatfoot in adults due to dysfunction of the posterior tibial tendon. J Bone Joint Surg Am 1999;81(8): 1173–82.
101. Soysa A, Hiller C, Refshauge K, et al. Importance and challenges of measuring intrinsic foot muscle strength. J Foot Ankle Res 2012;5(1):29–42.
102. Basmajian JV, Stecko G. The role of muscles in arch support of the foot: an electromyographic study. JBJS 1963;45(6):1184–90.
103. Farris DJ, Kelly LA, Cresswell AG, et al. The functional importance of human foot muscles for bipedal locomotion. Proc Natl Acad Sci U S A 2019;116(5):1645–50.
104. Headlee DL, Leonard JL, Hart JM, et al. Fatigue of the plantar intrinsic foot muscles increases navicular drop. J Electromyogr Kinesiol 2008;18(3):420–5.
105. Mulligan EP, Cook PG. Effect of plantar intrinsic muscle training on medial longitudinal arch morphology and dynamic function. Man Ther 2013;18(5):425–30.
106. Okamura K, Kanai S, Hasegawa M, et al. The effect of additional activation of the plantar intrinsic foot muscles on foot dynamics during gait. Foot (Edinb) 2018;34:1–5.
107. Franettovich Smith MM, Hides JA, Hodges PW, et al. Intrinsic foot muscle size can be measured reliably in weight bearing using ultrasound imaging. Gait Posture 2019;68:369–74.
108. Garofolini A, Taylor S, McLaughlin P, et al. Repeatability and accuracy of a foot muscle strength dynamometer. Med Eng Phys 2019;67:102–8.
109. Zhang X, Aeles J, Vanwanseele B. Comparison of foot muscle morphology and foot kinematics between recreational runners with normal feet and with asymptomatic over-pronated feet. Gait Posture 2017;54:290–4.

Update on Investigation Methods for Lower Extremity Biomechanics

John Tassone, DPM[a,b,*], Melanie Violand, DPM[c,1],
Evelyn G. Heigh, DPM, AACFAS[a,d], Chandler Hubbard, DPM[e],
Audris Tien, DPM[e], Jarrod Shapiro, DPM[f]

KEYWORDS

- Weight bearing computed tomography • Foot biomechanics • Radiographic angles
- MSK ultrasound

KEY POINTS

- Biomechanics of the foot is an essential component to the clinical podiatric assessment. Imaging augments and enhances the biomechanical examination.
- Plain film radiographs are the mainstay imaging used in biomechanics assessment. However, other imaging modalities are proving to be valuable in the biomechanical examination.
- Advanced imaging, such as weight bearing computed tomography scans and diagnostic ultrasound examinations, are emerging as valuable adjuncts to the biomechanical assessment.

INTRODUCTION

The combination of foot and ankle imaging and biomechanical assessment has been taught and written about for many years[1] and is widely used clinically, especially for surgical planning. Radiographs have been the mainstay of biomechanical analysis and are an excellent adjunct to the clinical biomechanical examination. Normal bony alignment with specific angles have been established and are used to

Disclosure Statement: The authors have nothing to disclose.
[a] Arizona School of Podiatric Medicine, Glendale, AZ, USA; [b] Private Practice, Summit Medical Group, Glendale, AZ, USA; [c] Arizona School of Podiatric Medicine, Midwestern University, Glendale, AZ, USA; [d] Private Practice, Summit Medical Group, 5620 West Thunderbird Road Suite G-2, Glendale, AZ 85306, USA; [e] Podiatric Medicine and Surgery with Rearfoot Reconstruction and Ankle Certificate, Chino Valley Medical Center, 5451 Walnut Avenue, Chino, CA 91710, USA; [f] PMSR/RRA Podiatric Residency, Western University College of Podiatric Medicine, Chino Valley Medical Center, 309 East Second Street, Pomona, CA 91766, USA
[1] Present address: 19955 North 59th Avenue, Glendale, AZ 85308.
* Corresponding author. 3415 East Kristal Way, Phoenix, AZ 85050.
E-mail address: jctassone@cox.net

Clin Podiatr Med Surg 37 (2020) 23–37
https://doi.org/10.1016/j.cpm.2019.08.003
0891-8422/20/© 2019 Elsevier Inc. All rights reserved.

podiatric.theclinics.com

adequately assess osseous alignment.[2] The purpose of using imaging with biomechanical analysis is to augment the clinical examination and improve outcomes by correlating imaging findings with the examination.

In addition to obtaining information about angular data and relational information, novel uses of imaging modalities have become increasingly common, especially pertaining to biomechanical studies. Modalities such as cone-beam weightbearing computed tomography (CT) scans and MRI have opened new avenues of biomechanical research and have helped to answer previously unanswered questions. They have also created new questions and controversies. Similarly, recent research using radiography have demonstrated notable pitfalls when interpreting these images.

This article reviews the use of modern imaging modalities as they are applied to biomechanics of the lower extremity. This discussion includes diagnostic musculoskeletal radiology as well as ultrasound examination, which helps to identify soft tissue pathology.[3] Other imaging such as MRI and CT scans are also discussed as a part of the changing paradigm in both the research realm as well as clinical environment. This article illustrates various uses of currently available imaging modalities in the biomechanical assessment of the lower limb with the goal of providing a more nuanced application of this technology.

IMAGING FUNDAMENTALS

A proper discussion of radiography must begin with a review of the 2 primary types of biomechanical data that may be obtained: kinematic and kinetic. As a review, kinematic data relate to positional information regarding bones and joints. For example, the position of one bone in relation to another during various aspects of the gait cycle provides kinematic data. Kinetics, in contrast, considers the forces acting on those bones and joints. The amount of force or pressure needed to cause rotation around the axis of a joint offers kinematic information. Static radiographs of the lower extremity have historically reported kinematic information. The reporting of kinetic data required technology outside of that used in lower extremity imaging with the important limitation that in vivo experiments were often not possible. Researchers were forced to rely on cadaveric methods to elucidate kinetic biomechanical information. This limitation has caused much of the surgical research to remain kinematic in nature, and surgeons were required to extrapolate postoperative normalization of abnormal bony angles and relationships to improvement of preoperative symptoms.

With the advent of modern biomechanical theories, imaging modalities have extended their usefulness in several ways. For example, one of the fundamental tenets of the tissue stress theory of biomechanical function is the identification of anatomic structures under tension.[4,5] The readily available use of MRI and ultrasound examination, for example, allows providers to noninvasively confirm specific damaged anatomy previously suspected during the physical examination. A damaged plantar metatarsophalangeal plate, for example, is more clearly visible on MRI or ultrasound examination and is impossible to directly visualize on radiographs. As a result of this improved understanding of the role of the plantar plate, a variety of novel surgical treatments have been invented to address this specific structure.[6–8] Similarly, MRI has greatly enhanced understanding of the role of the plantar calcaneonavicular spring ligament's role in the pathogenesis of adult acquired flatfoot deformity (AAFD).[9]

As a complement to the tissue stress theory, the subtalar axis location rotational equilibrium theory benefits from the kinematic understanding of foot function provided by static imaging. This theory allows for an estimation of the subtalar axis location and an extrapolation of the rotational forces acting on the foot, augmenting the physical examination.[10,11] This concept significantly adds to the planal dominance concept by combining older kinematic information with kinetic data for a more dynamic evaluation.

Radiographs for biomechanical purposes must be weightbearing.[12] Previously, only the dorsoplantar and lateral views were discussed because the angular measurements are not valuable assessments on oblique views.[13] However, newer radiographic views such as the long leg calcaneal axial[14] and hindfoot alignment views[15] assist in providing further information. Patients should stand in their angle and base of gait, because the goal is to capture the foot in its natural alignment during the active gait cycle.[16] Patients should also stand in the relaxed calcaneal stance position to indicate natural static positioning of joint alignment and pathology present without correction.[16] Each radiographic view allows an assessment of the plane orthogonal to that view. For example, the dorsoplantar view assesses the transverse axis of the foot and the lateral view assesses the sagittal plane.[16]

RADIOGRAPHY

Plain film radiography is the hallmark imaging modality used to evaluate angular relationships of the foot using various radiographic angles critical to determining foot pathology.[17,18] Specific normal values and pathologic measurement ranges are available in other resources.[17,18] This article updates the use of current imaging modalities for biomechanical assessment of the lower extremity.

There exists an intimate relationship between the talar declination angle, the calcaneal inclination angle, forefoot/metatarsus adductus, and the superimposition of the talus on the calcaneus. In a hyperpronated foot type, the talar declination angle is increased and the calcaneal inclination angle is decreased. The forefoot adductus decreases and the talus is less superimposed on the calcaneus. Hyperpronation leads to instability in the forefoot as well as the midfoot. Subluxation occurs and increases the forces leading to tissue strain. Radiographic assessment, coupled with clinical biomechanical findings, allows extrapolation of these abnormal forces and direct treatment to minimize them. Other radiographic findings associated with hyperpronation include an increased cuboid abduction angle, anterior breach of the cyma line, and an increase in the talocalcaneal angle on the dorsoplantar view (**Fig. 1**).

Specific foot types also have radiologic features that have a biomechanical correlation. A flexible forefoot valgus leads to late midstance subtalar joint pronation via supination of the longitudinal midtarsal joint axis. This appears as less superimposition of the talus on the calcaneus on the dorsoplantar radiograph. The calcaneal inclination

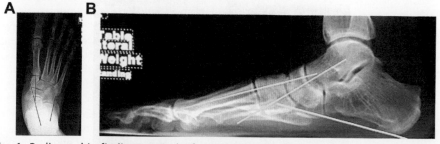

Fig. 1. Radiographic findings typical of pronation, including an increased talocalcaneal angle on both the dorsoplantar and lateral weightbearing views, increased talar declination, increased cuboid abduction, anterior cyma line break, decreased calcaneal inclination angle, and negative talofirst metatarsal angle.

angle may be high, and an elevated medial column owing to ground reactive forces inverting the forefoot may also be evident. Similarly, a compensated forefoot varus will lead to pronation at the subtalar joint, allowing the forefoot to invert relative to the ground. Ankle equinus deformity is often seen radiographically via its effect on mobile joints of the foot. This is demonstrated most apparently on the lateral radiograph of the Charcot neuroarthopathic foot with midfoot and forefoot dorsiflexion, typically at the location of the Charcot breakdown and a negative calcaneal inclination angle (**Fig. 2**). A similar, although less profound, effect is seen in the non-neuroarthropathic pes planus foot.

First ray and medial column function are critical for normal foot function. A plantar-flexed first ray, seen on the lateral radiograph, increases ground-reactive forces under the first ray leading to potential subtalar joint supinatory instability. Radiographic evaluation of the first ray and medial column have complexities that may affect clinical decision making and must be considered.

The Coleman block test was originally described to determine flexibility of the hindfoot in a pes cavus foot type with plantarflexed first ray.[19] During the examination, a block is placed under the forefoot, allowing the first metatarsal to hang without support. If the calcaneal bisection becomes rectus to the ground with the first ray off-loaded, then the varus heel is thought to be driven by the forefoot. This test may also be used radiographically to more accurately determine the change in hindfoot position with the first ray offloaded. Long leg calcaneal axial radiographs are obtained with the patient standing in the resting calcaneal stance position without the medial column offweighted and then again with a block under the lesser metatarsal heads. The tibiocalcaneal angle is measured in both instances and the difference between the 2 indicates the amount of reduction. This method has the ability to quantify the kinematic changes more accurately than the physical examination alone. A slight modification of the radiographic Coleman block test may also be performed in patients with a global anterior cavus deformity in which all metatarsals are plantarflexed, which may cause a compensatory rearfoot cavus. Standard radiographic lateral views demonstrate an increased calcaneal inclination angle. A second lateral radiograph is then obtained with the block offloading all 5 metatarsals. The calcaneal inclination angle is then remeasured and the difference between the 2 views indicates the total contribution of the forefoot equinus to the rearfoot cavus deformity (**Figs. 3** and **4**).

Radiographs also help to determine the location of medial column mobility. Originally, it was thought that medial column motion and increased mobility was located at the first metatarsocuneiform joint and was the primary indication for the Lapidus

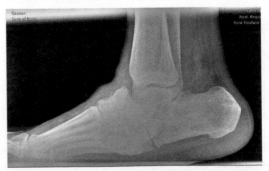

Fig. 2. Weightbearing lateral radiograph of a foot with lateral Lisfranc joint Charcot neuroarthropathy demonstrating relative forefoot dorsiflexion and functionally negative calcaneal inclination angle.

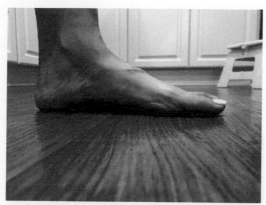

Fig. 3. Patient with subtle pes cavus deformity. Physical examination revealed an apparent global anterior cavus.

bunionectomy along with an adducted distal articular surface of the medial cuneiform.[20] This erroneous assumption may be demonstrated by comparing the clinical appearance of hallux limitus via the Hubscher maneuver (**Fig. 5**) with the corresponding weightbearing lateral radiograph (**Fig. 6**) showing elevation of the medial column at the naviculocuneiform joint (not the first tarsometatarsal joint) resulting in the limited first metatarsophalangeal joint motion seen in **Fig. 5**.

Recent research by Roling and colleagues[21] convincingly revealed the multijoint contribution to medial column motion with only an average 41% of sagittal motion measured at the first metatarsocuneiform joint, 50% of motion from the naviculocuneiform joint, and 9% from the talonavicular joint. This mixed contribution of motion was also noted by Phillips and colleagues[22] and Nester and colleagues.[23]

An additional pitfall has been noted when interpreting apparent medial column motion using the weightbearing lateral radiograph. Christman and colleagues[24] demonstrated that caution must be exercised when assessing metatarsus primus elevatus by means of the lateral radiographs alone as this finding may be artificially produced by altering the tube-head angulation and central beam direction. Using a standardized radiographic shadow system Christman found an apparent elevatus may be created with decreased tube head angulation and elevation. **Fig. 7** shows

A   **B**

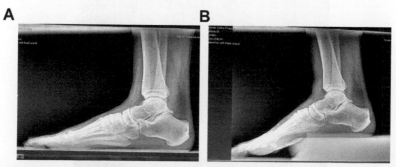

Fig. 4. Modification of the radiographic Coleman block test of the patient in **Fig. 3** to determine the contribution of a global anterior cavus to the rearfoot cavus. Note in this patient with a true rearfoot cavus the lack of change in the calcaneal inclination angle between the standard and forefoot offloaded views.

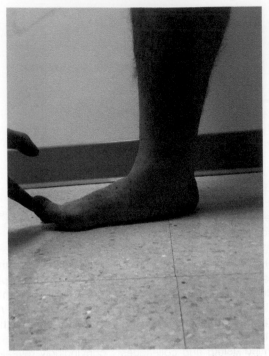

Fig. 5. Hubscher maneuver demonstrating the presence of hallux limitus with minimal hallux dorsiflexion and lack of arch raising effect.

lateral radiographs with 3 different tube-head angulations and the apparent metatarsus primus elevatus that becomes evident.

Just as a false elevatus may be created with variable tube-head angulation, so too may a radiographic atavistic cuneiform be an artifact. Sanicola and colleagues[25] found a discordance between the appearance of atavism and true atavism in the medial cuneiform. They radiographed a series of 515 random cadaver cuneiforms and first metatarsal bones to determine the angle of the distal articular surfaces of the medial

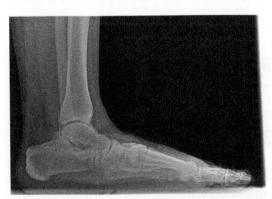

Fig. 6. Weightbearing lateral radiograph of the patient's foot from **Fig. 5** with no evidence of first tarsometatarsal mobility (no plantar gapping) and an absence of first metatarsal elevation. Dorsiflexion of the medial column is notable at the naviculocuneiform joint.

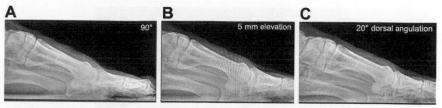

Fig. 7. Isolated forefoot weightbearing lateral radiographs demonstrating the creation of an apparent elevatus deformity with 2 different tube-head angulations.

cuneiforms. They found an apparent increase in the medial angulation of the medial cuneiform (creating a false atavistic appearance) when the first metatarsal was in an increased declination and inverted position. This false atavism was due to magnification of the dorsal ridge of the medial cuneiform. Similarly, Brage and colleagues[26] found the angle lessens significantly as the beam orientation changes from a 10° to a 30° tilt when studying 7 loaded cadaver feet. **Fig. 8** demonstrates this phenomenon in a single patient's dorsoplantar weightbearing radiograph. Sanicola and associated[25] recommend obtaining a weightbearing lateral radiograph from which the first metatarsal declination angle is measured. The central beam is the angled perpendicular to that measured angle rather than at the standard 15° cephalad to prevent evaluation errors.[25]

When reviewing the standard lateral radiograph, it is often difficult to determine which joint is contributing to the majority of motion of the medial column (**Fig. 9**). This is better clarified using radiographs in a more dynamic fashion. An additional modification to the radiographic Coleman block test has been described by Wood and colleagues,[27] called the reverse Coleman block test radiograph. This test is used to more accurately determine the level of medial column joint mobility in patients with flexible flatfoot conditions. In this test, a lateral radiograph is again obtained but with the block placed plantar to the first metatarsal head. The radiograph shows the location of the medial column motion (**Fig. 10**). Surgical or nonsurgical interventions may then be focused on the joint with the most motion.

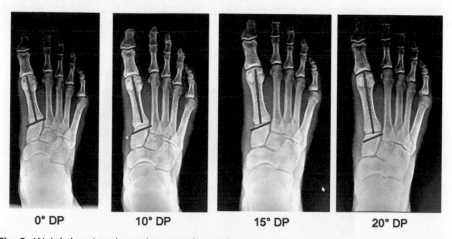

0° DP   10° DP   15° DP   20° DP

Fig. 8. Weightbearing dorsoplantar radiographic series of the same foot at different tube-head angulations. The oblique line at the first tarsometatarsal joint is at the same angle in all images and parallel to the line drawn at the far-left image. Note the decreased apparent atavism of the medial cuneiform with increased beam angulation.

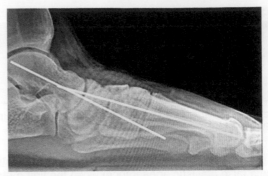

Fig. 9. Classic lateral radiograph. Note Meary's angle indicating a medial column breach closest to the talonavicular joint.

Radiographic measurements have also been used to predict posterior tibial tendon (PTT) tears. Calcaneal pitch may provide a strong association with injury to the supporting structures of the medial arch.[28] Lin and colleagues[28] found if both the calcaneal pitch and lateral talo-1st metatarsal (Meary's) angle were normal, no PTT tear was present. Additionally, a PTT tear was associated with abnormal talonavicular uncoverage angle, calcaneal pitch angle, Meary angle, and cuneiform-to-fifth metatarsal height. Conversely, if both the calcaneal pitch and Meary's angles were normal, no PTT tear was present. An abnormal calcaneal pitch angle had the best association with injury to the supporting medial longitudinal arch structures.

Recent controversy has erupted over the contribution of the frontal plane to hallux abductovalgus deformities. This debate has been spurred by the work of several researchers who have called into question the interpretation of previously considered standardized findings. Several authors have used the sesamoid axial radiograph to demonstrate pronation of the foot leading to a valgus rotation of the first metatarsal as well as valgus rotation of the sesamoids in hallux valgus deformities.[29–32] Dayton and colleagues[33] have argued that the increased tibial sesamoid position seen on the dorsoplantar radiograph is actually a sign of frontal plane rotation of the sesamoids. This phenomenon is demonstrated in **Fig. 11**. The sesamoids are everted in the sesamoid axial with the tibial sesamoid lateral to the bisection of the first metatarsal. This same lateralized appearance is also evident on the dorsoplantar radiograph of the same patient (central image, see **Fig. 11**).

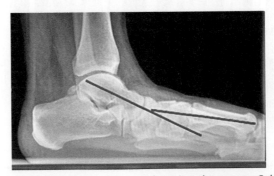

Fig. 10. Same patient's foot as in **Fig. 8** but undergoing the reverse Coleman block radiograph test. A paper wedge is under the first metatarsal head with medial column motion occurring at the naviculocuneiform joint, contrary to what is shown in **Fig. 9**.

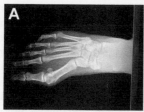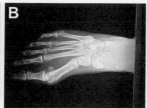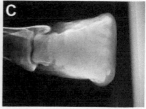

Fig. 11. Weightbearing dorsoplantar radiographs of normal (*A*) and frontal plane rotated (*B*, *C*) first metatarsals demonstrating lateral round sign, lateralized and externally rotated sesamoids, and laterally prominent first metatarsal base.

Okuda and colleagues[34] discussed lateral rounding of the first metatarsal head (positive round sign) seen in valgus metatarsal rotation and flattening of the first metatarsal head laterally after varus rotation of the first metatarsal (negative round sign). Similarly, Eustace and colleagues[35] found determination of frontal plane rotation was possible by examining the appearance of the inferior tuberosity of the first metatarsal base. With each 10° of first metatarsal rotation they found an increased laterality of the metatarsal base.[35] **Fig. 11** demonstrates these radiographic phenomena in 2 different feet, one with rotation of the first metatarsal and one without.

Some argument remains as to the overall validity of these methods. It has been pointed out that the sesamoid axial radiograph is not a true weightbearing study because the toes are dorsiflexed, and the patient is not standing in angle and base of gait. This dorsiflexed hallux position activates the windlass mechanism, which may cause the first metatarsal—and the attached sesamoids—to evert, creating what may seem to be an abnormal sesamoid position (Richie D. Personal communication, 2018). However, new weightbearing CT technology discussed elsewhere in this article sheds new light on this controversy.

MUSCULOSKELETAL ULTRASOUND EXAMINATION

Ultrasound examination is an excellent office-based imaging modality for diagnostic and therapeutic purposes when considering soft tissue injuries. However, there is a significant operator-dependent aspect to ultrasound imaging and a steep learning curve when first using the equipment. High-resolution ultrasound examination should be used to adequately assess soft tissue of the foot and ankle.[36] High resolution is defined as greater than 12 MHz, but it is more effective to use a resolution closer to an 18 MHz frequency.[37] This increase in direct and indirect axial resolution influences the lateral resolution of structures.

An advantage of ultrasound imaging is that it allows for dynamic assessment, which can be beneficial in identifying subtle injuries, such as minor tendon tears, subluxation of the peroneal tendons, and Haglund's deformity in which the pathology is related to mechanical irritation on the soft tissue during movement.[3] In fact, mechanical injury to the tendons and ligaments caused by bone hypertrophy needs the dynamic component that ultrasound provides. Ultrasound examination can also be used to specifically target an anatomic structure, which provides support to the tissue stress biomechanical theory in which the first step is to determine the injured or stressed anatomic structure.[4,5] Thus, ultrasound examination functions within the larger biomechanical paradigm and provides a fast and convenient way to assess biomechanical issues in real time and in dynamic fashion.

Ultrasound is also a valuable tool in assessing PTT dysfunction (PTTD). Ultrasound examination can be used to evaluate the PTT for peritendinitis, tenosynovitis, tendinosis, intrasubstance tears, and complete rupture. The ultrasound examination can evaluate tendon diameter, anatomy, and function during dynamic evaluation. The degree of tendinopathy can then be correlated with the clinical and radiographic findings to determine appropriate treatment.[38] Additionally, ultrasound examination can be used to evaluate the integrity of the spring ligament and the need for biomechanical control with nonsurgical or surgical treatment options.

Ultrasound examination also assists in identifying joint instability owing to plantar plate injuries or joint pathology by examining early erosive changes, and crystal deposition in joint effusion.[39] Angular abnormalities such as metatarsus adductus may necessitate increasing orthotic control owing to the increased pronatory force the angular abnormality creates.

MRI

As with musculoskeletal ultrasound examination, MRI may also contribute to biomechanical understanding by identifying injured anatomic structures. The best imaging of soft tissue structures is via MRI, and it should be used when suspicion of soft tissue injury requires clarification. Dislocations that cannot be detected by other modalities become easier to identify. MRI is specifically of value in low-grade Lisfranc injuries not identifiable by other means. MRI was found to be 94% sensitive and 75% specific for intraoperative stability.[40] Grading of ligamentous damage is possible. Identifying tendons (peroneus longus) caught in the dislocation that are likely to prevent conservative treatment from working is an added advantage of this technique. It must be noted that, like plain radiographs and CT scans, MRI is an examination performed on the unloaded foot, and some abnormalities may not be visible.

Similarly, MRI can accurately demonstrate altered anatomy of the spring ligament complex and deltoid ligament.[41,42] Spring ligament deformation precedes PTTD or AAFD. Specifically, MRI identifies spring ligament thickening or attenuation and partial tears. In PTTD, the PT tendon fails to invert the hindfoot and lock the transverse tarsal joint, causing the gastrocnemius–soleus complex to act at the talonavicular joint. Repetitive plantarward stress from the head of the talus leads to attenuation or tearing of the spring ligament with resultant plantarflexion of the talus, forefoot abduction and hindfoot valgus deformity.[43] In the future, understanding the extent of involvement of the spring ligament complex may provide prediction of success and failure of surgical and nonsurgical treatments.

MRI is also being explored to obtain kinematic evaluation of the foot. A promising early study validated the use of MRI to biomechanically study foot motion. They determined an end range of motion in various common positions and then built a custom device to hold living feet in 8 preassigned positions. Bone motion was quantified from maximum plantarflexion, inversion, and internal rotation to maximum dorsiflexion, eversion, and external rotation, which correlated well with previously published kinematic studies. This process offered a novel method to study foot biomechanical function.[44]

More recent studies with positional MRI have further identified potential usefulness. Positional MRI was performed in 10 healthy volunteers in supine, standing, standing with 10% load, and barefoot walking positions. The investigators measured movement of the navicular in 2 directions and compared the movement with stretch sensor measurements. They found good correlation of navicular movement to static stretch receptor measurements but were not able to predict dynamic movements with positional MRI.[45]

Probasco and colleagues[46] used weightbearing MRI to determine the orientation of the subtalar joint axis in patients with PTTD or AAFD after hypothesizing that these patients would have an increased valgus tilt of the subtalar joint itself. They examined 18 normal participants and 36 stage 2 patients with AAFD undergoing surgical reconstruction and found moderate to strong interrater and intrarater reliability for the use of this method. A more varus tilt of the subtalar joint articular surface in the normal patient control group and a valgus orientation of the joint surface in the AAFD patients were discovered. The study by Probasco and coworkers[46] study demonstrates the usefulness and future direction of biomechanical studies via 3-dimensional imaging technology, although there remain limitations to this technology, specifically by the inability to measure dynamic function and lack of kinetic data.

COMPUTED TOMOGRAPHY SCANS

As with standard radiographs, biomechanical measurements can be obtained from the weightbearing CT scan. Based on available literature, several measurements have been described to assess the forefoot alignment and midfoot–hindfoot alignment using the weightbearing CT scan.[47] The forefoot measurements include specifically assessment of hallux valgus deformity (α angle, hallux valgus angle, intermetatarsal angle, and tarsometatarsal angle). The hindfoot measurements include foot and ankle offset, hindfoot alignment angle, and osseous relationship (eg, talocalcaneal overlap and tibiocalcaneal distance).[47]

The weightbearing CT scan has been introduced as a potentially valuable tool that can provide functional information about joint biomechanics. A major limitation of conventional CT scans has been the inability to obtain weightbearing images. With weightbearing CT scans, true alignment of the lower extremity may be appreciated and pathology such as impingement, joint space narrowing, and malalignment that may be apparent only with load can be better understood.[47] The weightbearing CT scan is a rapidly developing technology derived from clinically established dental cone-beam scanners that can produce 300 images over a 210° projection angle with a total scan time of only 18 seconds.[48] Advantages of the novel portable cone-beam CT scanners include fast image acquisition time, high spatial resolution, imaging in the supine or physiologic standing position, and its small gantry size, make it practical and easily portable on its built-in wheels, with low radiation dose, and modest cost.[47,48] The clinical applications of weightbearing CT scan are far-reaching in lower extremity imaging and have only begun to be investigated in the mobility of the first ray as well as assessing syndesmotic stability after an ankle fracture, Lisfranc injury, and/or hindfoot alignment.

Collan and colleagues[49] performed a seminal study to determine if weightbearing CT scans could be used to measure frontal plane rotation of the metatarsals. They obtained weightbearing CT images of 10 patients with hallux valgus and 5 normal controls, recording the first intermetatarsal and hallux abductus angles. They also looked at rotation of the proximal hallux phalanx and first metatarsal in relation to ground. These researchers found a statistically significant eversion rotation of hallux proximal phalanx but not of the first metatarsal in comparison with controls. As a pilot investigational study one must be cautious when extrapolating results; this study had a small study size and unclear description of rotational and angular measurements. They did not measure or discuss sesamoid position, no measurements were made in comparison with the lesser metatarsals, and their reported results were not related to the stated purpose of the study.

In 2015, Kim and colleagues[50] performed a study examining sesamoid rotation using a new measurement method they termed the alpha (α) angle; this was a bisection of the tibial sesamoid position in relation to the weightbearing surface. Using semi-weightbearing CT axial images of 19 control feet without deformity compared with

166 feet with preoperative hallux valgus deformity, they found patients with hallux valgus had a greater incidence of pronated (externally rotated) first metatarsals. This study contradicted the results of the Kimura study, but it should be noted that both studies referenced coronal first metatarsal rotation with the weightbearing surface rather than the second metatarsal.

In 2017, Kimura and colleagues[51] studied the feet of 10 healthy patients with no history of foot pathology and 10 patients with severe hallux valgus deformity who were scheduled to undergo surgery. However, Kimura and colleagues did not use the cone-beam CT scan but rather created a loading device to be applied to the foot to reproduce a standing state while a conventional CT scanner was used (simulated but not true weightbearing). The 10 feet with hallux valgus deformity were compared with the normal feet, and the hallux valgus group also showed significantly greater dorsiflexion, inversion, and adduction of the first metatarsal relative to the medial cuneiform. In addition to finding hypermobility in the sagittal plane, feet with hallux valgus exhibited significantly more inversion and adduction at the first tarsometatarsal joint, which suggests that tarsometatarsal joint hypermobility involves motion in all 3 planes and at multiple joints of the medial column. Importantly, in reference to the frontal plane rotation in hallux valgus controversy, this study showed inversion of the first metatarsal rather than eversion in those patients with hallux valgus.

Considering Oldenbrook and Smith[30] in 1979 found valgus rotation of all 5 metatarsal heads during subtalar joint was pronation, it is unfortunate that these studies have chosen the weightbearing surface against which to compare rotation of the first metatarsal. This factor may be a significant reason for the variable outcomes and existence of this controversy. The authors of this article recommend studies adopt a protocol of full standing weightbearing CT images with comparison against both the ground and the second metatarsal.

As with the MRI studies described elsewhere in this article, multiplanar CT imagining may also be used to describe anatomy with potentially significant biomechanical effects. Cody and colleagues[52] reported using multiplanar CT to identify subtalar joint valgus in patients with adult acquired flatfoot. Another study by Kunas and colleagues[53] showed that, although CT imaging is valuable in assessing PTTD, multiplanar weightbearing imaging more effectively captures the amount of hindfoot valgus in full weightbearing stance. This modified CT measurement method is not widely available at this time and has a significant cost; thus, it is likely to remain in the academic environment for at least the near future.

SUMMARY

Biomechanical clinical assessment is seeing a renewal in novel uses of previously unconsidered imaging technology that has augmented and enhanced the uses of these imaging modalities. New uses of traditional radiography, ultrasonography examination, MRI, and CT scans have created new methods to research biomechanics in an increasingly dynamic way.

REFERENCES

1. Sgarlato TE. A compendium of podiatric biomechanics. San Francisco (CA): California College of Podiatric Medicine; 1971.

2. Kaschuk TJ, Layne W. Surgical radiology. Clin Podiatr Med Surg 1988;5(4):797.

3. Van Holsbeeck M, Introcaso JH. Musculoskeletal ultrasonagraphy. Mosby Year Book; 1991.

4. Mueller M, Maulf K. Tissue adaptation to physical stress: a proposed "physical stress theory" to guide physical therapist practice, education, and research. Phys Ther 2002;82(4):383–403.

5. McPoil T, Hunt G. Evaluation and management of foot and ankle disorders: present problems and future directions. J Orthop Sports Phys Ther 1995;21(6): 381–8.

6. Ford LA, Collins KB, Christensen JC. Stabilization of the subluxed second metatarsophalangeal joint: flexor tendon transfer versus primary repair of the plantar plate. J Foot Ankle Surg 1998;37(3):217–22.

7. Bouché RT, Heit EJ. Combined plantar plate and hammertoe repair with flexor digitorum longus tendon transfer for chronic, severe sagittal plane instability of the lesser metatarsophalangeal joints: preliminary observations. J Foot Ankle Surg 2008;47(2):125–37.

8. Sung W. Technique using interference fixation repair for plantar plate ligament disruption of lesser metatarsophalangeal joints. J Foot Ankle Surg 2015;54(3): 508–12.

9. Jennings M, Christensen J. The effects of sectioning the spring ligament on rearfoot stability and posterior tibial tendon efficiency. J Foot Ankle Surg 2008;47(3): 219–24.

10. Kirby K. Subtalar joint axis location and rotational Equilibrium theory of foot function. J Am Podiatr Med Assoc 2001;91(9):465–87.

11. Kirby K. Methods for determination of positional variations in the subtalar joint Axis. J Am Podiatr Med Assoc 1987;77(5):228 34.

12. Gamble FO. Yale I: clinical foot roentgenology. 2nd edition. Huntington (NY): Krieger Publishing; 1975.

13. Weissman SD. Radiology of the foot. Baltimore (MD): Williams and Wilkins; 1989.

14. Reilingh ML, Beimers L, Tuijthof GJ, et al. Measuring hindfoot alignment radiographically: the long axial view is more reliable than the hindfoot alignment view. Skeletal Radiol 2010;39:1103–8.

15. Saltzman C, El-Koury G. The hindfoot alignment view. Foot Ankle Int 1995;16(9): 572–6.

16. Weismann S. Standard radiographic techniques of the foot and ankle. Clin Podiatr Med Surg 1988;5(4):767–75.

17. Green DR. "Radiology and biomechanical foot types." reconstructive surgery of the foot and leg, Update'98. Tucker (GA): The Podiatry Institute; 1998. p. 292–315.

18. Lamm BM, Stasko PA, Gesheff MG, et al. Normal foot and ankle radiographic angles, measurements, and reference points. J Foot Ankle Surg 2016;55(5):991–8.

19. Coleman S, Chesnut W. A simple test for hindfoot flexibility in the cavovarus foot. Clin Orthop Relat Res 1977;123:60–2.

20. Lapidus PW. Operative correction of the metatarsus varus primus in hallux valgus. Surg Gynecol Obstet 1934;58:183–91, 16.

21. Roling B, Christensen J, Johnson C. Biomechanics of the first ray Part IV. The effect of selected medial column arthrodeses: a three-dimensional kinematic study on a cadaver model. J Foot Ankle Surg 2002;41(5):278–85.

22. Phillips RD, Law EA, Ward ED. Functional motion of the medial column joints of the foot during propulsion. J Am Podiatr Med Assoc 1996;86(10):474–86.

23. Nester CJ, Liu AM, Ward E, et al. In vitro study of foot kinematics using a dynamic walking cadaver model. J Biomech 2007;40(9):1927–37.

24. Christman RA, Flanigan KP, Sorrento DL, et al. Radiographic analysis of metatarsus primus elevatus: a preliminary study. J Am Podiatr Med Assoc 2001; 91(6):294–9.
25. Sanicola SM, Arnold TB, Osher L. Is the radiographic appearance of the hallucal tarsometatarsal joint representative of its true anatomical structure. J Am Podiatr Med Assoc 2002;92(9):491–8.
26. Brage ME, Holmes JR, Sangeorzan BJ. The influence of X-ray orientation on the first metatarsocuneiform joint angle. Foot Ankle Int 1994;15(9):495–7.
27. Wood EV, Syed A, Geary NP. Clinical tip: the reverse Coleman block test radiograph. Foot Ankle Int 2009;30(7):708–10.
28. Lin Y, Mhurircheartaigh J, Lamb J, et al. Imaging of the adult flatfoot: correlation of radiographic measurements with MRI. AJR Am J Roentgenol 2015;204:354–9.
29. Inman V. Hallux valgus: a review of etiologic factors. Orthop Clin North Am 1974; 5(1):59–66.
30. Oldenbrook L, Smith C. Metatarsal head motion secondary to rearfoot pronation and supination: an anatomical study. J Am Podiatry Assoc 1979;69(1):24–8.
31. Scranton P Jr, Rutkowski R. Anatomic variations in the first ray: part I. Anatomic aspects related to bunion surgery. Clin Orthop Relat Res 1980;151:244–55.
32. Scranton P Jr, Rutkowski R. Anatomic variations in the first ray: part II. Disorders of the sesamoids. Clin Orthop Relat Res 1980;151:256–64.
33. Dayton P, Kauwe M, Feilmeier M. Is our current paradigm for evaluation and management of the bunion deformity flawed? A discussion of procedure philosophy relative to anatomy. J Foot Ankle Surg 2015;54(1):102–11.
34. Okuda R, Yasuda T, Jotoku T, et al. Proximal abduction-supination osteotomy of the first metatarsal for adolescent hallux valgus: a preliminary report. J Orthop Sci 2013;18:419–25.
35. Eustace S, O'Byrne J, Stack J, et al. Radiographic features that enable assessment of first metatarsal rotation: the role of pronation in hallux valgus. Skeletal Radiol 1993;22(3):153–6.
36. Kremkau F. Diagnostic ultrasound, principals and instruments. 7th edition. St Louis (MO): Saunders; 2006.
37. Delzell P, Tritie B, Chiunda J, et al. Clinical utility of high frquency MSK ultrasonography: how ultrasound imaging influences diagnosis and treatment. J Foot Ankle Surg 2017;56(4):735–9.
38. Schumacher S. Sonographic imaging of the posterior tibial , flexor digitorum longus and flexor hallucis longus tendons. In: Tassone J, Barrett S, editors. Diagnostic ultrasound of the foot and ankle. Brooklandville (MD): Data Trace Publishing; 2015.
39. Borne J, Bordet B, Fantino O, et al. Plantar plate and second ray syndrome: normal and pathological US imaging features and proposed US classification. J Radiol 2010;91(5 Pt 1):543–8.
40. Raikin SM, Elias I, Dheer S, et al. Prediction of midfoot instability in the subtle Lisfranc injury: comparison of magnetic resonance imaging with intraoperative findings. J Bone Joint Surg Am 2009;91(4):892–9.
41. Chhabra A, Soldatos T, Chalian M, et al. 3-Tesla magnetic resonance imaging evaluation of posterior tibial tendon dysfunction with relevance to clinical staging. J Foot Ankle Surg 2011;50:320–8.
42. Chhabra A, Subhawong TK, Carrino JA. MR imaging of deltoid ligament pathologic findings and associated impingement syndromes. Radiographics 2010; 30:751–61.

43. Omar H, Saini V, Wadhwa V, et al. Spring ligament complex: illustrated normal anatomy and spectrum of pathologies on 3T MR imaging. Eur J Radiol 2016; 85(11):2133–43.

44. Fassbind MJ, Rohr ES, Hu Y, et al. Evaluating foot kinematics using magnetic resonance imaging: from maximum plantar flexion, inversion, and internal rotation to maximum dorsiflexion, eversion, and external rotation. J Biomech Eng 2011; 133(10):104502.

45. Johannsen F, Hansen P, Stallknecht S, et al. Can positional MRI predict dynamic changes in the medial plantar arch? An exploratory pilot study. J Foot Ankle Res 2016;9(35):1–8.

46. Probasco W, Haleem AM, Yu J, et al. Assessment of coronal plane subtalar joint alignment in peritalar subluxation via weight-bearing multiplanar imaging. Foot Ankle Int 2015;36(3):302–9.

47. Barg A, Bailey T, Richter M, et al. Weightbearing computed tomography of the foot and ankle: emerging technology topical review. Foot Ankle Int 2018;39(3): 376–86.

48. Tuominen EK, Kankare J, Koskinen SK, et al. Weight-bearing CT imaging of the lower extremity. AJR Am J Roentgenol 2013;200(1):146–8.

49. Collan L, Kankare JA, Mattila K. The biomechanics of the first metatarsal bone in hallux valgus: a preliminary study utilizing a weight bearing extremity CT. Foot Ankle Surg 2013;19(3):155–61.

50. Kim Y, Kim JS, Young KW, et al. A new measure of tibial sesamoid position in hallux valgus in relation to the coronal rotation of the first metatarsal in CT scans. Foot Ankle Int 2015;36(8):944–52.

51. Kimura T, Kubota M, Taguchi T, et al. Evaluation of first-ray mobility in patients with hallux valgus using weight-bearing CT and a 3-D analysis system. J Bone Joint Surg Am 2017;99-A(3):247–55.

52. Cody EA, Williamson ER, Burket JC, et al. Correlation of talar anatomy and subtalar joint alignment on weightbearing computed tomography with radiographic flatfoot parameters. Foot Ankle Int 2016;37(8):874–81.

53. Kunas GC, Probasco W, Haleem AM, et al. Evaluation of peritalar subluxation in adult acquired flatfoot deformity using computed tomography and weightbearing multiplanar imaging. Foot Ankle Surg 2018;24:495–500.

Medial Column Biomechanics
Nonsurgical and Surgical Implications

Francis Chan, DPM[a],*, Melinda A. Bowlby, DPM[b,c,1],
Jeffrey C. Christensen, DPM[b,c,1]

KEYWORDS

- Medial column • Biomechanics • Windlass • First ray • Hallux valgus • Flatfoot

KEY POINTS

- The medial column is composed of dynamic and static stabilizers. Dynamic stabilizers consist of the windlass mechanism and peroneus longus locking mechanism. Dysfunction of the dynamic as well as the static stabilizers of the medial column plays a role in pathomechanics.
- Conservative options for addressing the medial column include custom foot orthotics and bracing.
- Options for addressing the medial column surgically include first tarsometatarsal joint arthrodesis, opening plantarflexory medial cuneiform osteotomy, and naviculocuneiform arthrodesis with the goal to restore the stable tripod configuration.

INTRODUCTION

A true understanding of medial column biomechanics is paramount to a successful outcome whether treating a patient conservatively or after hallux valgus or flatfoot surgery. There are several seemingly dogmatic classification systems that exist for the flatfoot; however, each flatfoot presents in a unique way and several factors must be taken into account.[1] Dysfunction of the dynamic as well as the static stabilizers of the medial column play a role in pathomechanics. The presence of first ray insufficiency, forefoot varus, first ray elevatus, naviculocuneiform faulting, and an associated bunion deformity must be identified. The presence of equinus, which acts as a deforming force on the medial column, must also be assessed.

[a] Private Practice, 5000 Kingsway, Suite #320, Burnaby, BC V5H 2E4, Canada; [b] Department of Orthopedics, Swedish Medical Center, Seattle, WA, USA; [c] Department of Orthopedics, Providence Medical Center, Everett, WA, USA
[1] Present address: 3131 Nassau St, Suite #101, Everett WA, 98201.
* Corresponding author.
E-mail address: fc@fcfootandankle.com

Clin Podiatr Med Surg 37 (2020) 39–51
https://doi.org/10.1016/j.cpm.2019.08.004
0891-8422/20/© 2019 Elsevier Inc. All rights reserved.

DYNAMIC STABILIZATION OF THE MEDIAL COLUMN AND PATHOGENESIS OF THE WINDLASS MECHANISM

The windlass mechanism was first described by Hicks.[2] He found the plantar aponeurosis is composed of 3 bands, with the central band attaching to the sesamoid bones, plantar plates of the lesser metatarsals, plantar fat pad, and skin of the forefoot. Hicks[2] observed that, with extension of the hallux, the plantar aponeurosis shortens and he provided the analogy of hallux extension as the action of winding up a cable: the plantar aponeurosis (**Fig. 1**). The winding up of the plantar aponeurosis then creates a shortened foot, raised arch, supinated hindfoot, and externally rotated leg. It is the central band that provides the greatest arch-raising effect in the windlass mechanism.[2–5] This mechanism helps to convert the foot into a rigid lever in late stance, in preparation for toe-off.

The cablelike winding of the plantar aponeurosis is analogous to a spring with the ability to store strain energy, stabilize the arch, and release the energy in an elastic recoil.[6] Thordarson and colleagues[7] sequentially transected the plantar aponeurosis in cadavers and measured the changes in fascial band length and arch height in a closed kinetic chain. They confirmed the dynamic shortening effect and the arch-raising effect of an activated plantar aponeurosis with maximal hallux extension. The windlass mechanism has also been indirectly observed in a kinematic study.[8] During gait, the foot lengthens in the first 50% of the stance phase, then the foot starts shortening at midstance with arch raising, reaching maximum arch height at 80% of stance phase just after heel-off. With increased walking speed, foot shortening and arch-raising effects became more augmented, showing the windlass mechanism and the foot's ability to adapt its stability for different speeds.[8]

The effectiveness of the windlass mechanism relies on appropriate alignment of its osseous attachments.[9] Rush and colleagues[9] loaded cadaver limbs and measured first ray motion with abnormal first metatarsal and sesamoid alignment, and compared it with corrected first metatarsal and sesamoid alignment. With an increased intermetatarsal 1-2 angle and laterally deviated sesamoids, the first ray sagittal plane motion was the same regardless of whether the hallux was plantigrade or placed in maximal dorsiflexion.

Interestingly, once the intermetatarsal 1-2 angle and sesamoid positions were corrected, first metatarsal plantarflexion was found to be significantly different with the hallux placed in maximal extension compared with first ray plantarflexion with hallux in plantigrade position. Similar significant results were seen with the medial cuneiform

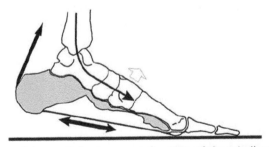

Fig. 1. A rigid beam of the medial column as a function of the windlass mechanism and a stable first ray. Load can pass through the first ray as the entire forefoot shares in the load transmission. (*From* Morton DJ. Metatarsus atavicus. The Identification of a Distinct Type of Foot Disorder. *J Bone Joint Surg.* 1927;9–A:531–544; with permission.)

sagittal plane position when first metatarsal and sesamoids were corrected, and when the windlass mechanism was activated. The study confirmed that the windlass action effectively raised the arch by increasing the first ray plantarflexion by 26%.[9] This concept is further supported by Coughlin and colleagues[10] in a study of cadaveric specimens with a hallux valgus deformity. A proximal crescentic osteotomy and a distal soft tissue reconstruction was performed, which resulted in a mean decrease in intermetatarsal angle from 12.9° to 6.8°.[10] The first ray sagittal motion was also decreased from a mean of 11 mm to 5.2 mm.[10] Therefore, restoring the first ray to near-normal anatomy allows the windlass mechanism to function efficiently to provide first ray stability.[10]

In hallux valgus surgery, improper realignment of the sesamoids underneath the first metatarsal has contributed to early recurrence of hallux valgus deformity.[11,12] With the sesamoids subluxed from the first metatarsosesamoidal articulation, hallux extension may not be able to activate the windlass mechanism for meaningful arch raising and foot shortening stabilization through first ray plantarflexion. Consequently, with one of the dynamic stabilizing mechanisms of the medial column functioning suboptimally, more reliance is placed on the remaining dynamic and static stabilization mechanisms. Over time, the remaining stabilizers may fail.

PERONEUS LONGUS LOCKING MECHANISM

Duchenne[13] observed the agonist-antagonist relationships between the peroneus longus, tibialis anterior, and tibialis posterior on the position of the first ray. When the function of peroneus longus is lost, the tibialis anterior function became unopposed, resulting in gradual elevation of the first metatarsal and development of flatfoot.[13] Peroneus longus has been identified to be active in midstance and heel-off during gait.[14]

Johnson and Christensen[15] later confirmed Bohne's[16] finding of peroneus longus function to resist first metatarsal medial deviation. Johnson and Christensen[15] axially loaded cadaveric feet and loaded midstance tendons while measuring the positional changes of the first metatarsal, medial cuneiform, navicular, and talus with varying peroneus longus strengths. With increasing strength of the peroneus longus in closed kinetic chain, the first metatarsal and medial cuneiform became more everted and plantarflexed (**Fig. 2**). More proximal effects to the navicular were also observed, with the navicular everting and dorsiflexing with increasing peroneus longus load. The multiplanar effect of peroneus longus in closed kinetic chain on the first metatarsal, medial cuneiform, and navicular positions were all significant.

Perez and colleagues[17] furthered research the peroneus longus locking mechanism by simulating different frontal plane positions to evaluate its effect on sagittal plane motion of the first ray. With the first metatarsal held in maximum everted position, simulating a peroneus longus locking mechanism, the first ray dorsal excursion was significantly less than when the first metatarsal was in neutral position at the first metatarsocuneiform joint (**Fig. 3**). In contrast, with the first metatarsal held in maximum inversion, simulating a metatarsus primus varus, the first ray dorsal excursion was significantly elevated compared with when the first ray was in neutral position.

Dullaert and colleagues[18] later confirmed these findings via a closed kinetic chain, cadaveric study with computed tomography scan imaging to evaluate positional changes of medial column bones with a flaccid peroneus longus and with a loaded

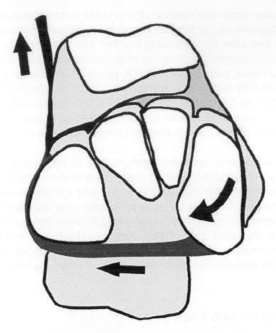

Fig. 2. Cross section through the midfoot along with the distal course of the peroneus longus. Note the torsional lever arm of the medial cuneiform with the action of the peroneus longus and the wedge shape of the intermediate cuneiform, which can control dorsal migration of the first ray. (*From* Morton DJ. Metatarsus atavicus. The Identification of a Distinct Type of Foot Disorder. *J Bone Joint Surg.* 1927;9–A:531–544; with permission.)

peroneus longus. The first metatarsal everted significantly with peroneus longus pull, and interestingly, the first and second intermetatarsal angles decreased under these conditions too. They did not find more proximal medial column effects from the peroneus longus as was found in Johnson and Christensen's[15] study, which might be because of the peroneus longus tendon being loaded in isolation without loading other active, midstance tendons.

Duchenne was[13] the first to identify the agonist-antagonist relationship between the peroneus longus and triceps surae. The contributing effect of equinus on forefoot pain, plantar fasciitis, Achilles tendonitis, and flatfoot conditions have been well accepted. Isolated gastrocnemius equinus being a contributor to isolated forefoot and midfoot pain in the absence of hindfoot deformity has been confirmed.[19] DiGiovanni and colleagues[19] found that patients who had isolated forefoot and midfoot pain had an average maximal ankle dorsiflexion of 4.5° with knee extension, whereas the control group had an average maximal ankle dorsiflexion of 13.1° with knee extension. Differences in ankle dorsiflexion with extended knee were found to be significant between these two groups. When ankle dorsiflexion was measured with the knee in flexion, the significant difference was no longer appreciated between the two groups. In the final study of a biomechanics research series, Johnson and Christensen[20] provided a greater understanding of biomechanical effects of equinus on the medial column. With increasing Achilles tendon load in closed kinetic chain, the first metatarsal became significantly inverted, showing the opposing effect of equinus to the eversion pull of the peroneus longus.[20]

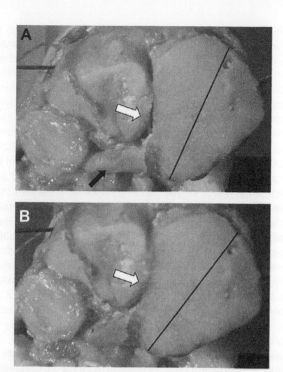

Fig. 3. Gross anatomic specimen cut at the proximal metatarsals. (*A*) The first ray is in neutral position. Note the space between the first and second ray resembling an open packed or unlocked position. The insertion of peroneus longus (*black arrow*); note the oblique course. (*B*) The first ray is in an everted position. Note the lack of space and tight fit resembling a closed packed or locked position (*white arrow*). In addition, note the plantar lateral shelf of the first ray under-riding the second ray. (*From* Perez HR, Reber LK, Christensen JC. The Effect of Frontal Plane Position on First Ray Motion: Forefoot Locking Mechanism. Foot Ankle Int. 2008;29:72–76; with permission.)

STATIC STABILIZATION OF THE MEDIAL COLUMN AND PATHOGENESIS

Morton[21] was the first to describe hypermobility of the first metatarsal, which was defined as an increase in dorsal movement or hyperextension of the first metatarsal bone, resulting in lowering or collapse of the medial arch with weight bearing. He attributed this excessive dorsal excursion to a slack first metatarsocuneiform ligament, relative to the other plantar ligaments of the second through fifth tarsometatarsal joints. Consequently, lesser metatarsals would have to bear more of the weight-bearing load and could contribute to lesser metatarsal overload. Morton[22] also observed similar symptoms in feet with shortened first metatarsals. The stability at the first metatarsocuneiform joint and the length of the first metatarsal helps maintain the rigid lever function in the forefoot for force transmission through gait. The loss of either of the aforementioned static stabilization characteristics of the first ray is termed first ray insufficiency.[23]

Since Morton's[21,22] description, numerous studies have attempted to define hypermobility of the first ray by quantifying it.[4,24,25] Klaue and Hansen[24] developed a device that helped to measure the amount of first metatarsal dorsal excursion, and the Klaue device has been validated for its accuracy and provides interobserver and intraobserver reliability.[24,26] Despite having this tool, a quantitative definition has yet to be determined. Traditional manual examination for first ray hypermobility is not a reliable method for measuring hypermobility in isolation. An alternative manual examination, described as the windlass activation test, to the traditional manual examination for dorsal excursion at the first tarsometatarsal joint was offered by Christensen and Jennings.[23] The windlass activation test evaluates the first tarsometatarsal joint dorsal excursion while accounting for the patient's static stabilization and dynamic stabilization from the windlass mechanism (**Fig. 4**). This modified manual examination may allow examiners to better understand each patient's first ray biomechanics.

Variations to the first metatarsal proximal articular facets may also provide some insight on the function of the first ray. Morton[22] and Lapidus[27] thought that the oblique medial cuneiform and first metatarsal joint was an atavistic trait that was responsible for the development of the hallux valgus deformity. Normal variations in articular facets have been identified.[28,29] Mason and Tanaka[28] found that, when a proximal first metatarsal articular surface is made of a unifacet or a bifacet, it was more likely to present in feet with hallux valgus. When a trifacet was seen at the first metatarsal proximal articular surface, it was never present in feet with hallux valgus. The unifacet and bifacet may be an anatomic indicator for first ray hypermobility, and the trifacet may indicate a more structurally stable joint orientation.[28] Doty and colleagues[30] found that continuous facets were associated with a higher intermetatarsal angle but that neither the contour of the facets nor the degree of the medial inclination correlated with hypermobility. In addition, they found that the suggested atavistic medial cuneiform is a product of radiographic beam angle.

The naviculocuneiform joint also contributes to first ray and medial column biomechanics.[31,32] Roling and colleagues[31] simulated fusions in cadaveric feet without deformity, at the metatarsocuneiform joint, naviculocuneiform joint, and talonavicular joint separately, to find the contribution of first ray range of motion from these joints. The metatarsocuneiform, naviculocuneiform, and talonavicular joints provided 41%, 50%, and 9% of first ray range of motion, respectively. However, the difference in the amount of first ray range of motion contributed by the metatarsocuneiform and naviculocuneiform fusions was not statistically different.

Furthermore, each joint fusion had no significant impact on the range of motion of the unfused medial column joints. This finding supports Hansen's[33] theory that the first metatarsocuneiform joint and the naviculocuneiform joints are unnecessary joints of

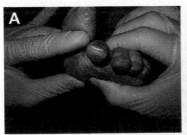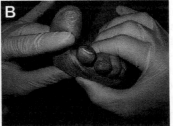

Fig. 4. A patient who had severe subsecond metatarsalgia after fascia release and over-lengthening. There is no evidence of first ray hypermobility and metatarsals I and II are of equal length and declination. The windlass activation test was performed and revealed there was persistent first ray mobility with the windlass engaged, explaining the metatarsalgia. Lack of dynamic load sharing of the first and second metatarsals was confirmed with pedobarographic testing. (*A*) Starting position after windlass activation. (*B*) First ray elevates with manual testing. (*From* Morton DJ. Metatarsus atavicus. The Identification of a Distinct Type of Foot Disorder. *J Bone Joint Surg.* 1927;9–A:531–544; with permission.)

the foot, because simulated fusion of these joints did not significantly affect the motion of the other joints. Hansen[33] theorized that certain joint motions within the foot do not contribute to the range of motion that is essential or important for gait; therefore, fusion of the unnecessary joints does not limit the function of the foot postoperatively.

NONSURGICAL IMPLICATIONS

Custom foot orthotics have been the mainstay in conservative care; however, there is a lack of consensus in the literature from biomechanical and clinical research for the use of custom foot orthotics. One reason for this may be that kinematic studies can be highly variable and difficult to design. Nonetheless, the authors often prescribe custom foot orthotics before surgery as well as postoperatively for their patients. Orthotics can help stabilize the medial column by preloading the plantar fascia and maintaining first ray plantarflexion.[34] Forefoot posting can also be useful to support a forefoot varus. Not all patients tolerate an orthotic device, especially as the deformity progresses. Custom ankle foot orthotics may be useful at this point in the case of advanced adult acquired flatfoot for patients who are not surgical candidates. Little can be done to strengthen an insufficient medial column in the way of physical therapy. When equinus coexists with medial column pathomechanics or medial column deformity, regular calf stretching exercises are recommended. However, it remains unproved that gastrocnemius and soleus stretching can be beneficial for a pathologic medial column.

SURGICAL IMPLICATIONS

The medial and lateral columns may only be treated as separate entities when independent movement exists between them. If the adult acquired flatfoot has progressed to a rigid, fixed deformity, then a reverse Cole-type transtarsal osteotomy is needed to realign the foot. Most commonly, medial column procedures are combined in conjunction with either a gastrocnemius recession and/or posterior tibial tendon repair if these disorders are also present. Medial column procedures may also be combined with lateral column lengthening and calcaneal column osteotomies when necessary with the goal to restore a stable tripod configuration. Options for addressing the medial column include first tarsometatarsal joint arthrodesis, opening plantarflexory medial cuneiform osteotomy (Cotton osteotomy), and naviculocuneiform arthrodesis.

FIRST TARSOMETATARSAL JOINT ARTHRODESIS

The Lapidus bunionectomy, first described in 1934, has now become one of the most indispensable procedures in foot and ankle surgery.[35] The first tarsometatarsal joint arthrodesis is the logical choice for medial column stabilization in skeletally mature patients with first ray insufficiency. Recently, frontal plane malalignment of the first metatarsal in hallux valgus deformity has gained attention. Dayton and colleagues[36] showed that, as the valgus rotation of the first metatarsal increases, so does the tibial sesamoid position and the intermetatarsal angle. Therefore, applying a varus force to the first metatarsal to reduce intermetatarsal angle has been observed to reduce the tibial sesamoid position.[36,37] An intraoperative reduction technique has been described by DiDomenico and colleagues[37] in which a varus thrust is applied to the hallux to correct the frontal plane, the hallux is dorsiflexed to correct the sagittal plane, and medial pressure is applied to the first metatarsal head to correct the transverse plane.

Even in the absence of a bunion deformity, an arthrodesis of the first tarsometatarsal joint is often performed in lieu of a naviculocuneiform arthrodesis, in order to provide medial column stability, if there is minimal peritalar subluxation and naviculocuneiform faulting (**Fig. 5**). The first tarsometatarsal joint arthrodesis has the benefit of correcting first ray insufficiency and hallux valgus, and also enhances medial column stability.[9,38] The increase in medial column support was observed in increases to the talo-first metatarsal angle and the medial cuneiform height, after the Lapidus arthrodesis.[39] Catanzariti and colleagues[40] described, and Bierman and colleagues[38] later confirmed, the stabilizing effect of the first tarsometatarsal joint arthrodesis on the medial column by increasing the efficiency of the peroneus longus tendon.

Much to the surgeon's chagrin, as potentially a reason for the recurrence of hallux valgus after Lapidus bunionectomy, intercuneiform instability continues to be poorly understood. In an attempt to diagnose the condition, a fluoroscopic splay test, in which the surgeon's thumb and forefinger exert pressure between the first and second metatarsal heads, has been described.[41] If there is residual splay of the first metatarsal, the consideration of fixation between the first and second metatarsal bases is recommended.[41] Roling and colleagues[31] observed the greatest reduction in first ray range of motion with simulated Lapidus arthrodesis with intercuneiform arthrodesis, compared with isolated first tarsometatarsal joint arthrodesis or naviculocuneiform arthrodesis.

Anecdotally, the authors have noticed fractures of the second metatarsal base with fixation between the first and second metatarsal bases. The authors' preferred approach to treat intercuneiform instability is the use of first metatarsal to intermediate cuneiform fixation or intercuneiform fixation. The sagittal first ray hypermobility can be further reduced with the addition of first metatarsal to intermediate cuneiform fixation.[42] The nonunion rate for the first tarsometatarsal joint ranges

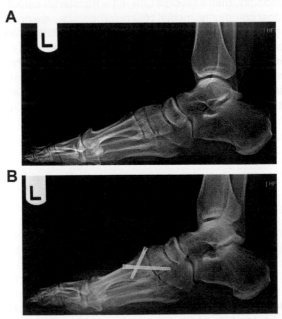

Fig. 5. (*A*) Preoperative lateral radiograph. Note the first ray elevatus and naviculocuneiform fault. (*B*) Postoperative lateral radiograph after a first tarsometatarsal joint arthrodesis. The first ray elevatus is corrected, naviculocuneiform fault is reversed, and the subtalar joint is supinated.

in the literature from 3.3% to 12%, although joint preparation and fixation vary widely among reports.[43] Although not yet proved, the additional use of first metatarsal to intermediate cuneiform fixation is thought to result in a stronger surgical construct and may decrease the rate of nonunions (Vickers M, personal communication. Seattle, WA 2019).

COTTON OSTEOTOMY

In 1936, Cotton[44] originally described a medial cuneiform osteotomy with a plantarflexory bone graft for an elevated first ray that helped rebalance the foot and restore the foot's tripod configuration.[45] Cotton osteotomy can be a useful procedure to realign the medial column in both pediatric and adult acquired flatfoot.[45] It also improves medial column stability by increasing first ray plantarflexion and the tension on the plantar fascia, thereby improving the effect of the windlass mechanism.[45] In the absence of hypermobility, an increased intermetatarsal angle, a naviculocuneiform fault, or osteoarthritis, a Cotton osteotomy is an ideal procedure.[45] The Cotton procedure is generally well tolerated and there are 2 articles that report a delayed union; however, to the authors' knowledge, nonunions have not been reported in the literature.[45,46]

NAVICULOCUNEIFORM ARTHRODESIS

The naviculocuneiform arthrodesis is the procedure of choice to stabilize the hypermobile medial column with a naviculocuneiform fault and to correct forefoot varus in adult acquired flatfoot. A plantar and medial wedge can be removed, thereby improving the sagittal and transverse plane deformities, providing the same effect as lateral column lengthening while only addressing the medial column.[47] Peritalar subluxation, Meary angle, and calcaneal inclination can be improved with the naviculocuneiform arthrodesis[43,48,49] (Fig. 6). Forefoot abduction and forefoot varus develop as the spring ligament and posterior tibial tendon begin to attenuate, and deformity of the rearfoot may soon follow.[50] Greisberg and colleagues[43,49] introduced the concept of forefoot-driven rearfoot valgus and proposed that medial column insufficiency may be the cause of peritalar subluxation, and that stabilizing the medial column acts as a post and reduces talar uncovering.

In severe cases, subtalar and talonavicular arthrodesis alone do not correct forefoot varus. It is prudent to consent the patient for a naviculocuneiform arthrodesis when performing a combined subtalar and talonavicular joint arthrodesis, which, if necessary, can be performed to correct any residual forefoot varus at the end of the surgery. Engaging the windlass mechanism is a useful maneuver in surgery to provide manual reduction of the naviculocuneiform joints before placement of fixation.[47] Although the naviculocuneiform arthrodesis is a powerful procedure that can realign the rearfoot while sparing essential joints, nonunion rates have been reported as high as 12.5%.[48,49]

COMBINED FIRST TARSOMETATARSAL JOINT AND NAVICULOCUNEIFORM JOINT ARTHRODESIS

In 1927, Miller[51] described the combined first tarsometatarsal joint and naviculocuneiform arthrodesis.[52] A combined first tarsometatarsal joint and naviculocuneiform joint fusion is usually performed in cases of long-standing medial column instability that has resulted in osteoarthritis of both joints. In these cases, arthrodesis of both joints cannot be avoided.

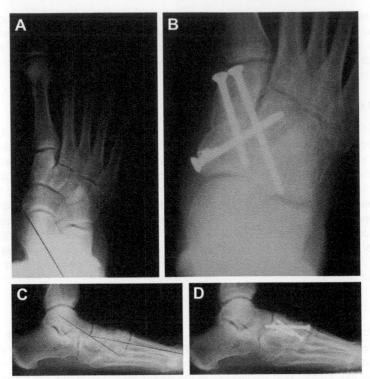

Fig. 6. (*A*) Preoperative anteroposterior radiograph. Note the peritalar subluxation. (*B*) Postoperative anteroposterior radiograph after a naviculocuneiform joint arthrodesis with improved peritalar subluxation. (*C*) Preoperative lateral radiograph. Note the decreased calcaneal inclination angle and increased Meary angle. (*D*) Postoperative lateral radiograph after a naviculocuneiform joint arthrodesis with improved Meary angle and calcaneal inclination angle.

However, clinicians must be cautious of iatrogenically creating an excessively rigid medial column that will be both poorly tolerated by the patient and result in adjacent joint osteoarthritis in the future.[1] As previously mentioned, Roling and colleagues[31] determined that arthrodesis of the first tarsometatarsal joint limits first ray sagittal plane range of motion by 41% and that naviculocuneiform arthrodesis limits first ray sagittal plane range of motion by 50%, which, combined, would reduce range of motion by a total of 91%. Furthermore, the combined first tarsometatarsal joint and talonavicular joint holds a nonunion rate that has been documented as high as 15%.[49,53]

COMBINED NAVICULOCUNEIFORM AND SUBTALAR ARTHRODESIS

There are some situations, especially in advanced adult acquired flatfoot, in which subtalar joint arthrodesis may be used to correct rearfoot valgus and naviculocuneiform joint arthrodesis may be used to correct forefoot varus and abduction, thereby sparing the talonavicular joint but still achieving triplanar correction. With this approach, peritalar subluxation can be improved as well as the biomechanics of the first ray.[52] Barg and colleagues[52] described a combined subtalar and naviculocuneiform arthrodesis in a small case series with positive results. Combined arthrodesis of the first tarsometatarsal joint, naviculocuneiform joint, and talonavicular joint can achieve more stability and lead to a more effective correction, which is often necessary.[52] However, the advantage of sparing the talonavicular joint, when possible, may reduce stress on adjacent joints and decrease the development of osteoarthritis.[52]

SUMMARY

A careful biomechanical and radiographic examination is a crucial part of preoperative planning in order to avoid undercorrecting as well as creating an overly rigid medial column. The presence of first ray insufficiency, forefoot varus, first ray elevatus, naviculocuneiform faulting, and an associated bunion deformity must be identified. The presence of equinus, which acts as a deforming force on the medial column, must also be assessed. Once the medial column biomechanical disorder is determined, several surgical options exist, including a first tarsometatarsal joint arthrodesis, opening plantarflexory medial cuneiform osteotomy (Cotton osteotomy), and naviculocuneiform arthrodesis. When addressing the medial column surgically, clinicians must have a flexible intraoperative plan with the end goal to restore a stable tripod configuration. In addition, diagnostic criteria for the hypermobile first ray and intercuneiform instability remain largely unknown and are 2 areas that require future investigation.

REFERENCES

1. Kadakia A, Kelikian A, Barbosa M. Did failure occur because of medial column instability that was not recognized, or did it develop after surgery? Foot Ankle Clin N Am 2017;22:545 62.
2. Hicks JH. The mechanics of the foot. II The plantar aponeurosis and the arch. J Anat 1954;88:25–31.
3. Bojsen-Møller F, Flagstad KE. Plantar aponeurosis and internal architecture of the ball of the foot. J Anat 1976;121:599–611.
4. Mizel MS. The role of the plantar first metatarsal first cuneiform ligament in weight bearing on the first metatarsal. Foot Ankle 1993;14:82–4.
5. Kitaoka HB, Luo ZP, Growney ES, et al. Material properties of the plantar aponeurosis. Foot Ankle Int 1994;15:557–60.
6. Ker RF, Bennett WB, Bibbyt SR, et al. The spring in the arch of the human foot. Nature 1987;325:147–9.
7. Thordarson DB, Kumar PJ, Hedman TP, et al. Effect of partial versus complete plantar fasciotomy on the windlass mechanism. Foot Ankle Int 1997;18:16–20.
8. Stolwijk NM, Koenraadt KLM, Louwerens JWK, et al. Foot lengthening and shortening during gait: a parameter to investigate foot function? Gait Posture 2014;39: 773–7.
9. Rush SM, Christensen JC, Johnson CH. Biomechanics of the first ray. Part II: metatarsus primus varus as a cause of hypermobility. A three-dimensional kinematic analysis in a cadaver model. J Foot Ankle Surg 2000;39(2):68–77.
10. Coughlin MJ, Jones CP, Valadot R, et al. Hallux valgus and first ray mobility: a cadaveric study. Foot Ankle Int 2004;25:537–44.
11. Okuda R, Kinoshita M, Yasuda T, et al. Postoperative incomplete reduction of the sesamoids as a risk factor for recurrence of hallux valgus. J Bone Joint Surg Am 2009;91-A:1637–45.
12. Ray RG. First metatarsocuneiform arthrodesis: technical consideration and technique modification. J Foot Ankle Surg 2002;41:260–72.
13. Duchenne GB. Physiologie des Mouvements. Paris: Bailliere; 1949 (Translated to: Physiology of Motion). Philadelphia: J. B. Lippincott Co.

14. Gray EG, Basmajian JV. Electromyography and cinematography of leg and foot (normal and flat) during walking. Anat Rec 1968;161:1–16.
15. Johnson CH, Christensen JC. Biomechanics of the first ray. Part I. The effects of peroneus longus function: a three-dimensional kinematic study on a cadaver model. J Foot Ankle Surg 1999;38(5):313–21.
16. Bohne WHO. Action of the peroneus longus tendon on the first metatarsal against metatarsus primus varus force. Foot Ankle Int 1997;18:510–2.
17. Perez HR, Reber LK, Christensen JC. The effect of frontal plane position on first ray motion: forefoot locking mechanism. Foot Ankle Int 2008;29:72–6.
18. Dullaert K, Hagen J, Klos K, et al. The influence of the Peroneus Longus muscle on the foot under axial loading: a CT evaluated dynamic cadaveric model study. Clin Biomech 2016;34:7–11.
19. DiGiovanni CW, Kuo R, Tejwani N, et al. Isolated gastrocnemius tightness. J Bone Joint Surg Am 2002;84-A:962–70.
20. Johnson CH, Christensen JC. Biomechanics of the first ray part V: the effect of equinus deformity. A 3-dimensional kinematic study on a cadaver model. J Foot Ankle Surg 2005;44(2):114–20.
21. Morton DJ. Hypermobility of the first metatarsal bone: the interlinking factor between metatarsalgia and longitudinal arch strains. J Bone Joint Surg 1928;10: 187–96.
22. Morton DJ. Metatarsus atavicus. The identification of a distinct type of foot disorder. J Bone Joint Surg 1927;9-A:531–44.
23. Christensen JC, Jennings MM. Normal and abnormal function of the first ray. Clin Podiatr Med Surg 2009;26:355–71.
24. Klaue K, Hansen ST Jr, Masquelet AC. Clinical, quantitative assessment of first tarsometatarsal mobility in the sagittal plane and its relation to hallux valgus deformity. Foot Ankle 1994;15:9–13.
25. Wanivenhaus A, Pretterklieber M. First tarsometatarsal joint: anatomical biomechanical study. Foot Ankle 1989;9:153–7.
26. Jones CP, Coughlin MJ, Pierce-Villadot R, et al. The validity and reliability of the Klaue device. Foot Ankle Int 2005;26:951–6.
27. Lapidus P. Operative correction of the metatarsus varus primus in hallux valgus. Surg Gynecol Obstet 1934;58:183.
28. Mason LW, Tanaka H. The first tarsometatarsal joint and its association with hallux valgus. Bone Joint Res 2012;1:99–103.
29. Hyer CF, Philbin TM, Berlet GC, et al. The incidence of the intermetatarsal facet of the first metatarsal and its relationship to metatarsus primus varus: a cadaveric study. J Foot Ankle Surg 2005;44:200–2.
30. Doty JF, Coughlin MJ, Hirose CB, et al. First metatarsocuneiform joint mobility: radiographic, anatomic, and clinical characteristics of the articular surface. Foot Ankle Int 2014;35:504–11.
31. Roling BA, Christensen JC, Johnson CH. Biomechanics of the first ray. Part IV: the effect of selected medial column arthrodeses. A three-dimensional kinematic analysis in a cadaver model. J Foot Ankle Surg 2002;41(5):278–85.
32. Faber FWM, Kleinrensink GJ, Verhoog MW, et al. Mobility of the first tarsometatarsal joint in relation to hallux valgus deformity: anatomical and biomechanical aspects. Foot Ankle Int 1999;20:651–6.
33. Hansen ST Jr. Functional reconstruction of the foot and ankle. 1st edition. Philadelphia: Lippincott Williams & Wilkins; 2000.
34. Scherer PR. Recent advances in orthotic therapy: improving clinical outcomes with a pathology-specific approach. Lower Extremity Review LLC.; 2011.

35. McCormick JJ, Johnson JE. Medial column procedures in the correction of adult acquired flatfoot deformity. Foot Ankle Clin N Am 2012;17:283–98.
36. Dayton P, Feilmeier M, Hirschi J, et al. Observed changes in radiographic measurements of the first ray after frontal plane rotation of the first metatarsal in a cadaveric foot model. J Foot Ankle Surg 2014;53:274–8.
37. DiDomenico LA, Fahim R, Rollandini J, et al. Correction of frontal plane rotation of sesamoid apparatus during the Lapidus procedure: a novel approach. J Foot Ankle Surg 2014;53:248–51.
38. Bierman RA, Christensen JC, Johnson CH. Biomechanics of the first ray. Part III. Consequences of Lapidus arthrodesis on peroneus longus function: a three-dimensional kinematic analysis in a cadaver model. J Foot Ankle Surg 2001; 40(3):125–31.
39. Avino A, Patel S, Hamilton GA, et al. The effect of the Lapidus arthrodesis on the medial longitudinal arch: a radiographic review. J Foot Ankle Surg 2008;47: 510–4.
40. Catanzariti AR, Mendocino RW, Lee ML, et al. The modified Lapidus arthrodesis: a retrospective analysis. J Foot Ankle Surg 1999;38:322–32.
41. Weber AK, Hatch DJ, Jensen JL. Use of the first ray splay test to assess transverse plane instability before first metatarsocuneiform fusion. J Foot Ankle Surg 2006;45:278–82.
42. Galli MM, McAlister JE, Berlet GC, et al. Enhanced Lapidus arthrodesis: crossed screw technique with middle cuneiform fixation further reduces sagittal mobility. J Foot Ankle Surg 2015;54(3):437–40.
43. Jordan TH, Rush SM, Hamilton GA, et al. Radiographic outcomes of adult acquired flatfoot corrected by medial column arthrodesis with or without a medializing calcaneal osteotomy. J Foot Ankle Res 2011;50:176–81.
44. Cotton FJ. Foot statistics and surgery. N Engl J Med 1936;214:353–62.
45. Boffeli TJ, Schnell KR. Cotton osteotomy in flatfoot reconstruction: a review of consecutive cases. J Foot Ankle Surg 2017;56(5):990–5.
46. Hirose CB, Johnson JE. Plantarflexion opening wedge medial cuneiform osteotomy for correction of fixed forefoot varus associated with flatfoot deformity. Foot Ankle Int 2004;25(8):568–74.
47. Ford LA, Hamilton GA. Naviculocuneiform arthrodesis. Clin Podiatr Med Surg 2004;21(1):141–56.
48. Gerrity M, Williams M. Naviculocuneiform arthrodesis in adult flatfoot: a case series. J Foot Ankle Surg 2019;58(2):352–6.
49. Greisberg J, Assal M, Hansen ST Jr, et al. Isolated medial column stabilization improves alignment in adult-acquired flatfoot. Clin Orthop Relat Res 2005;435: 197–202.
50. Castaneda D, Thordarson DB, Charlton TP. Radiographic assessment of medial cuneiform opening wedge osteotomy for flatfoot correction. Foot Ankle Int 2012;33:498–500.
51. Miller O. A plastic foot operation. J Bone Joint Surg 1927;9:84–91.
52. Barg A, Brunner S, Zwicky L, et al. Subtalar and naviculocuneiform fusion for extended breakdown of the medial arch. Foot Ankle Clin 2011;16(1):69–81.
53. Metzl JA. Naviculocuneiform sag in the acquired flatfoot: what to do. Foot Ankle Clin 2017;22(3):529–44.

The Lateral Column

Beth Jarrett, DPM, CPed[a],*, Timothy Cheung, MS, CPT[b],
Elizabeth Oh, BS, CPT[c]

KEYWORDS

- Fifth ray • Calcaneocuboid joint • Lateral column function • Biomechanics
- Arch collapse • Low gear • High gear

KEY POINTS

- The lateral column is a major functional unit within the foot as it relates to lower extremity biomechanics, consisting of the calcaneus, cuboid, fourth and fifth rays, and the corresponding phalanges.
- Of these structures, the fifth ray and calcaneocuboid joint complex are the major functional components.
- Dysfunction in lateral column kinematics can lead to pathology.
- The state of the field requires more evidence to appropriately assess the true role of lateral column biomechanics and function within the foot and lower extremity.

INTRODUCTION

Lower extremity biomechanics is the cornerstone of podiatric medicine and surgery. Indeed, the foot and ankle act as the interface between the ground and the proximal segments, acting to dynamically balance ground reaction forces (GRFs) and external moments with the body's internal moments. In most feet, GRFs act lateral to the subtalar joint axis, producing a pronatory torque until rotational equilibrium is met.[1–3] Although the medial and longitudinal arches of the foot produce load-sharing capabilities, the internal moments required to obtain rotational equilibrium can be overwhelmed by excessive GRFs, leading to late stance phase pronation and hypermobility.[4] Conversely, in some cases, the foot is rigid and unable to locally distribute lateral GRFs across an area, leading to pressure accumulation at the point of contact, the lateral column.[5,6] Although the medial longitudinal arch has been widely

Disclosure Statement: The authors have nothing to disclose.
[a] Dr. William M. Scholl College of Podiatric Medicine, Rosalind Franklin University of Medicine and Science, 3333 Green Bay Road, North Chicago, IL 60064-3095, USA; [b] Dr. William M. Scholl College of Podiatric Medicine, School of Graduate and Postdoctoral Studies, Rosalind Franklin University of Medicine and Science, 3333 Green Bay Road, North Chicago, IL 60064, USA; [c] College of Podiatric Medicine, Western University of Health Sciences, 309 E. Second Street, Pomona, CA 91766, USA
* Corresponding author.
E-mail address: beth.jarrett@rosalindfranklin.edu

researched, the details of the lateral longitudinal arch are less extensively delineated. The purpose of this review is to analyze the biomechanics of the lateral column as it relates to lower extremity function.

STRUCTURE AND FUNCTION OF THE LATERAL COLUMN

The lateral column consists of the calcaneus, cuboid, fourth and fifth rays, and the corresponding phalanges. Of these structures, the fifth ray and the calcaneocuboid joint (CCJ) complex are the major functional components. The fifth ray, or fifth metatarsal, is the most lateral component of the forefoot and the point at which GRF acts in low-gear walking, described by Bojsen-Møller as the use of the oblique axis of the metatarsophalangeal joints during propulsion.[7] Importantly, fifth ray anatomy and its theoretic axis of motion are well accepted. The fifth ray rotates about a triplanar axis oriented from posterior inferolateral to anterior superomedial, permitting pronation and supination.[8,9] The fifth ray has the ability to distribute or absorb GRF, and the ability of the fifth ray to pronate and supinate is speculated to correlate with its ability to distribute shock.[10] Thus, any disturbance in fifth ray motion during gait is hypothesized to disrupt its ability to manage the effects of GRFs.

To illustrate the function of the fifth ray on lateral column and lower extremity function, specific anatomic structures that are directly related to pathology within the lateral column are discussed.[11,12] The most notable characteristic of the fifth ray structure is its specialized base region, which is particularly important as it relates to its soft tissue attachments. The posterior surface of the base is triangular in shape as it articulates with the lateral apex of the cuboid. The medial surface of the base has a smooth facet reserved for the fourth ray articulation. The lateral surface of the base contains a relatively large tuberosity, the styloid process, which serves as the site of insertion for the peroneus brevis tendon, whereas the dorsal surface of the base provides a stable lever for the peroneus tertius tendon. Plantarly, the base of the fifth ray serves as an attachment for the long plantar ligament and the origins of the flexor digiti minimi brevis. The inferomedial surfaces of the base and shaft provide a site of origination for the third plantar interosseous muscle, and the superomedial surface serves as the origin for the fourth dorsal interosseous muscle.

The shaft and head of the fifth ray mimic the characteristics seen in other metatarsals. The shaft tapers from base to head, with a plantar concave curvature. Interestingly, Fallat and Buckholz[13] observed a lateral angulation of the head to its shaft in relationship to tailor's bunionette. Furthermore, Crawford contributed a radiographic technique to identify the apex of the lateral bowing.[14]

Distally, the fifth ray articulates with the base of the proximal phalanx. Similar to the first ray, the fifth ray was expected to benefit from Hicks'[15] proposed windlass mechanism, due to the slips of plantar aponeurosis that insert into the plantar plates. Bojsen-Møller unveiled the complexity of the lateral column, however, specifically at the CCJ; it became loose-packed in a simulated low-gear position, inhibiting the lateral column from experiencing the retrograde plantarflexion at its distal portlon.[7] Moreover, this lack of windlass effect seemed to be related to the radius of the metatarsal heads, of which the fifth ray's was smaller than that of the first ray. Thus, dorsiflexion at the metatarsophalangeal joint provides retrograde plantarflexion of the first ray and assists in supination of the subtalar joint, whereas the midtarsal joint is maximally pronated but not the fifth ray.[10] Distally, the interphalangeal joints hold negligible effects on the lateral column. The fifth distal interphalangeal joint is the most common coalition in the foot, at approximately 30%, yet usually remains asymptomatic.[16]

The structure of the CCJ is concavoconvex, with the articulating surface of the cuboid described as similar to the end of an hour glass with processes that extend dorsolaterally and inferiorly as a tongue-like projection. The articulating surface of the calcaneus reflects a congruent surface that complements the adjoining end of the cuboid to a high degree. The structure allows the cuboid to rotate on the calcaneus and pivot along the calcaneal process with some gliding motion available on the joint periphery. The main axis of the CCJ runs in a longitudinal direction with a secondary axis located through the lateral body of the calcaneus in a superomedial direction.

During high-gear push off, pronation of the forefoot with respect to the hindfoot occurs, resulting in the CCJ to be closely packed. With stabilization of the transverse tarsal joints, the foot becomes a rigid lever for propulsion and allows the longitudinal arch to stabilize preventing midtarsal break. In addition, the transverse metatarsophalangeal axis migrates to the region near the great toe and the ball of the foot. With low-gear push off, the forefoot inverts relative to the rearfoot and, as a result, the CCJ becomes loosely packed. Pressures are then more localized postaxially across the lateral region of the foot. The axis is transferred toward the lateral region of the submetatarsal heads. Subsequently, the lateral toes are forced into dorsiflexion with the hallux stabilizing the medial region.

A study by Greiner and Ball[17] investigated the mobility of the CCJ, concluding that the rotation of the cuboid in response to inversion-eversion forces of the forefoot was as high as 25° about an oblique axis. On the contrary, Blackwood and colleagues[18] noted no significant cuboid frontal plane motion in response to forefoot dorsiflexion, plantarflexion, inversion, and eversion while the calcaneus is everted and inverted. These reported variations may point to the adaptability of the CCJ and lateral column, but there remains a lack of sufficient evidence.

OPEN QUESTIONS ABOUT THE LATERAL COLUMN

The current knowledge of lateral column anatomy and function has facilitated treatment decisions for clinical management and surgical corrections. Indeed, current knowledge of the lateral column is necessary, yet incomplete. For instance, there still are no reliable estimates in the literature regarding fifth ray range of motion. If available, this information could be used to approximate moment arms of different forces that act around the lateral column determining the magnitude of torque to ultimately analyze motion and static equilibrium. Furthermore, arthrokinematic investigation of the fifth ray during specific activities, such as walking or running, will provide a holistic understanding of lateral column function. For example, the fifth ray does not solely pronate and supinate. Its motion also depends on the gliding and rolling at the tarsometatarsal joint.

Classically, it was believed that joints were restricted to 3 planes of motion: sagittal, frontal, and/or transverse motions. This theory was based on an older doctrine, however, that assumed a fixed axis of rotation. Now, it is widely accepted that the axis of rotation in a joint is shifted when the joint undergoes arthrokinematic motions: roll, glide, and spin.[19] Furthermore, the instantaneous shift in position of the axis can now be estimated, based on the motion and geometry of the articular surfaces.[20] For instance, the fifth metatarsocuboid joint is a synovial joint that is classically uniaxial and triplanar, deviating 20° from the transverse plane, 35° from the sagittal plane, and 70° from the frontal plane, permitting pronation and supination.[8,9] Because the articulating surface of the proximal fifth ray is slightly concave and the lateral facet of the distal cuboid is slightly convex, the fifth ray also utilizes arthrokinematic motion. Thus, this proximal articulation introduces a functional anatomy concept: the convex-concave rule, which describes the rolling and gliding arthrokinematics motions of a joint.[19] The concept states that if a concave articulating surface moves on a convex surface, the gliding and rolling occur in the same direction. Conversely, if the convex articulating surface moves on a concave surface, the rolling and gliding motions are opposite directions. Further investigation may demystify the lateral column as it relates to function and biomechanics.

Further complicating the concept are the subtalar and midtarsal joints. According to Elftman,[21] the midtarsal joint axes become more parallel (more motion) or more deviated (less motion), depending on the position of the subtalar joint. If motion is available at the CCJ, the cuboid cannot be considered the stationary limb, at least until it has reached its end range of motion. As a result, fifth ray motion will be affected. The shift of fifth tarsometatarsal joint axis position due to arthrokinematic motion requires further exploration. Human and cadaveric experiments that quantify the motion of the fifth ray while controlling the motion of the cuboid without interfering with the rest of the foot, similar to those demonstrated by Blackwood and colleagues,[18] would help decipher the differences between isolated fifth ray and lateral column ranges of motion.[22] Moreover, it would be interesting to retrospectively analyze patients with isolated calcaneocuboid arthrodesis and observe changes in gait pattern to elucidate the effects of CCJ obliteration on the fifth ray and lateral column. Revealing the role that these arthrokinematic motions have on the lateral column may have an important contribution in appropriately treating patients.

THERE ARE MULTIPLE APPROACHES TO DEMONSTRATING LATERAL COLUMN FUNCTION

Although the anatomy of the lateral column is widely accepted, its function as an independent unit or contribution to lower extremity function has yet to be clearly defined. Despite an abundance of case studies and small research projects on surgical fixations of fractured fifth rays, the knowledge of fifth ray function on the lateral column remains incomplete. This deficit can be detrimental to the clinical decision-making process, further emphasizing the importance of producing strong research about the lateral column.

Fortunately, speculations of lateral column functions can be made when considering the components of locomotion. Generally, Perry and Burnfield[23] describe 4 major components of locomotion: energy conservation, shock absorption, stance stability, and propulsion. Specifically, by using normal gait parameters as a model, it may be possible to interpolate the functions of the lateral column within lower extremity biomechanics.

Energy Conservation

Energy can be measured by many different routes. A common technique used by biomechanists is the manipulation of inverse dynamics. Mass and acceleration of movements are measured to calculate force, which can be further manipulated into various calculatable parameters.[24] One of the calculatable parameters is power (P). Power is the product of torque (τ) and angular velocity (ω) (Equation 1).

$$P = \tau * \omega \tag{1}$$

Conventionally, when power is positive, it indicates that a muscle is concentrically contracting and mechanical energy is generated. Conversely, when the power is negative, it indicates that a muscle is eccentrically contracting and mechanical energy is absorbed.[25] By collimating attention to the foot and ankle, it was able to be understood that the energy conservation and generation are balanced. The one issue, or 28 issues, with this model, is that many global models represent the foot and ankle as a unisegmental model. Foot and ankle specialists understand that the foot does not act as a single long bone on a single hinge to the leg by the ankle. Rather, it behaves in a coordinated and complex pattern. Thus, what is to prevent the progression of lateral column research from being studied in a similar manner? Major tendons that support the lateral column belong to the 3 peroneal muscles, 2 of which conveniently insert onto the base of the fifth ray and the last providing suspensory support to the cuboid.[11] Furthermore, multisegmental motion analysis of the foot and ankle, coupled with electromyographic (EMG) studies, may help elucidate the complex components of the lateral column function in energy conservation.

Stability

Another component of gait is stability, the ability to maintain static equilibrium in a dynamic environment or the ability to maintain a relative position in space while in motion. Often, stability is threatened by external and internal perturbations, such as GRFs, momentum, and muscular imbalances. Moreover, fifth ray and calcaneocuboid instability can manifest as lateral foot pain.[26] Indirectly, instability at other joints can lead to lateral column pathology. For instance, the lateral ankle sprain is one of the most frequent athletic injuries in the foot and ankle.[27] In patients with chronic ankle instability, the peroneals are thought to compensate, which can lead to an overuse injury.[28] Specifically, the peroneus brevis inserts at the styloid process of the base of the fifth ray, providing plantarflexion and eccentric pronation of the fifth ray. If the integrity of peroneus brevis is attenuated, the ability to eccentrically pronate the fifth ray may be dissipated, followed by a mitigated ability to absorb shock (discussed later), resulting in fractures or hypermobility. Moreover, the peroneus longus uses the peroneal sulcus of the cuboid as a pulley to eccentrically control first ray motion. Peroneus longus pathology may disrupt the cuboid pulley system, causing suboptimal function, such as that in cuboid syndrome and first ray hypermobility. Thus, identifying any relationships between lateral column stability and function relative to pathology is critical.

Propulsion and Shock Absorption

Operationally, propulsion may be defined as the ability to generate force to launch the body forward, whereas shock absorption is the ability to dissipate the forces acted on the body. Naturally, these two components of gait are antagonistic. In our field, imbalance of propulsion and shock absorption is commonly related to first ray (first metatarsal, first cuneiform, and all associated joints) pathology. A common manifestation of first ray imbalance of propulsion and shock absorption can be referred to as first ray hypermobility, debatably a state in which the first ray is in an unstable position when it should be stable. This manifestation is well known to have relationships with numerous pathologies associated with it.[29–35] Literature describing a possible hypermobile fifth ray remains incomplete, however, especially in the context of an unstable CCJ.

$$Mechanical\ Shock = Force = mass * acceleration \qquad (2A)$$

$$Force = \frac{mass * velocity}{time} \qquad (2B)$$

$$Force = \frac{momentum}{time} \qquad (2C)$$

If shock absorption is the ability to dissipate the amount of force applied to the body, then derivation of the shock equation (Equations 2A, B) reveals its two basic components: momentum and time (Equation 2C). Momentum can be altered by extrinsic factors. An example of how this translates into podiatry is the use of a medial rearfoot wedge to match an isolated rearfoot varus in an attempt to decrease pronatory momentum. On the contrary, the time of force application can be controlled intrinsically or extrinsically. Extrinsically, gymnasts tumble on specific mats that provide a cushion for landing.[36] The cushion increases the time between initial contact with the mat to the point of complete stop of downward motion. But intrinsically, highly trained gymnasts eccentrically flex their hips and knees while dorsiflexing their ankles and, pronating their feet as they land, extending the time of force application to allow for force dissipation.[37,38] Both of these mechanisms increase the time it takes to reach the end motion, thereby absorbing the high magnitudes of repetitive shock, such as in gait. This concept can be translated into gait mechanics at the lateral column. Because stiffness has a negative effect on shock absorption, the rigid lateral column of the foot must have an important effect in the foot's ability to absorb shock.[38]

Under normal conditions of the loading phase of gait, the lateral column collapses in response to pronatory effects of GRFs. But anything that limits these motions during the loading phase can impair shock absorption (ie, arthritis, arthrodesis, and narrow toe box in shoes). Furthermore, there is an intricate balance between shock absorption and propulsion. Not surprisingly, this balance has a temporal relationship. Propulsion requires the lateral column to be stable in order to act as a rigid lever whereas an unstable lateral column is required for shock absorption. A stable lateral column, assuming controlled midfoot and rearfoot stability, allows for the axis of rotation to transition from the ankle to the metatarsophalangeal joints during the propulsive phase of gait. There may be situations, however, when the fifth ray or CCJ is still unstable to absorb shock while the rest of the foot is transitioning into propulsion. It is critical to identify the relationship between specific areas within lateral column instability as it relates to late pronation and hypermobility. This area requires further investigation to identify the biomechanical implications of a hypermobile lateral column, an unstable lateral column that is required to be stable. Moreover, it can be speculated that the lack of shock absorption capabilities by the lateral column can lead to mechanical deterioration, such as fractures. Motion analysis studies, coupled with EMG studies and pressure-plate analyses, may provide further insight of the lateral column function in shock absorption and propulsion.

SUMMARY

The lateral column is one of the most important components of the foot, playing a significant role in lower extremity function. Moreover, dysfunction in lateral column kinematics is directly related to pathology. Although much of its biomechanics and contribution to the lateral column can be speculated through contemporary biomechanical theories, the state of the field requires more evidence to appropriately assess the true role of lateral column biomechanics and function within the foot and lower extremity.

REFERENCES

1. Donatelli RA. Normal biomechanics of the foot and ankle. J Orthop Sports Phys Ther 1985;7(3):91–5.

2. Kirby K. Biomechanics of normal and abnormal foot. J Am Podiatr Med Assoc 2000;90(1):30–4. Available at: https://pdfs.semanticscholar.org/6421/ 88e5644c3e1cd7f75e5f92010282214f8462.pdf.

3. Kirby KA. Subtalar joint axis location and rotational equilibrium theory of foot function. J Am Podiatr Med Assoc 2014;91(9):465–87.

4. Kirby KA. Longitudinal arch load-sharing system of the foot. Rev Española Podol 2017;28(1):e18–26.

5. Williams D III, McClay I, Hamill J, et al. Lower extremity kinematic and kinetic differences in runners with high and low arches. J Appl Biomech 2001;17:153–63.

6. Grech C, Formosa C, Gatt A. Shock attenuation properties at heel strike: implications for the clinical management of the cavus foot. J Orthop 2016;13(3):148–51.

7. Bojsen-Møller F. Calcaneocuboid joint and stability of the longitudinal arch of the foot at high and low gear push off. J Anat 1979;129(Pt 1):165–76. Available at: http://www.ncbi.nlm.nih.gov/pubmed/511760%0Ahttp://www.pubmedcentral.nih. gov/articlerender.fcgi?artid=PMC1233091.

8. Valmassy R. Clinical biomechanics of the lower extremities. 1st edition. Mosby; 1996.

9. Levangie PK, Norkin CC. Joint structure and function: a comprehensive analysis. 5th edition. F.A. Davis Company; 2011.

10. Caravaggi P, Pataky T, Günther M, et al. Dynamics of longitudinal arch support in relation to walking speed: contribution of the plantar aponeurosis. J Anat 2010; 217(3):254–61.

11. Netter F. The CIBA collection of medical illustrations: part 1 volume 8 musculoskeletal system. CIBA Pharmaceutical Company; 1977.

12. Standring S. Gray's anatomy. 41st edition. Elsevier; 2015.

13. Fallat L, Buckholz J. An analysis of the Tailor's bunion by radiographic and anatomical display. J Am Podiatr Med Assoc 1980;70(12):597–603.

14. Dunn SP, Pontious J. Tailor's Bunion Deformity. In: Southerland JT, editor. McGlamry's Comprehensive Textbook of Foot and Ankle Surgery. 4th edition. Wolters Kluwer/Lippincott Williams & Wilkins Health; 2013. p. 235–44.

15. Hicks JH. The mechanics of the foot: plantar aponeurosis and the arch. J Anat 1954;88(1):25–31.

16. Buyuk AF, Ozcan C, Camurcu Y, et al. The incidence of biphalangeal fifth toe: comparison of normal population and patients with foot deformity. J Orthop Surg 2019;27(1). 230949901982552.

17. Greiner TM, Ball KA. The calcaneocuboid joint moves with three degrees of freedom 2008;2:1–2.

18. Blackwood CB, Yuen TJ, Sangeorzan BJ, et al. The midtarsal joint locking mechanism. Foot Ankle Int 2005;26(12):1074–80. Available at: papers://eb2db329- 465b-4791-b47f-c3347d944097/Paper/p128.

19. MacConaill M. The movements of bones and joints: the significance of shape. J Bone Joint Surg Br 1953;35B(2):290–7.

20. Moorehead JD, Montgomery SC, Harvey DM. Instant center of rotation estimation using the Reuleaux technique and a Lateral Extrapolation technique. J Biomech 2003;36(9):1301–7.

21. Elftman H. The transverse tarsal joint and its control. Clin Orthop 1960;16:41–6.

22. Park DS, Schram AJ, Stone NM. Isolated lateral tarsometatarsal joint arthrodesis: a case report. J Foot Ankle Surg 2000;39(4):239–43.

23. Perry J, Burnfield J. Gait analysis: normal and pathological function. J Sports Sci Med 2010;9(2):353.

24. Robertson DGE. Research methods in biomechanics. 2004 2013. p. 309. Available at: http://books.google.com/books?id=oWVYeMiX4rMC&pgis=1.
25. Robertson G, Winter D. Mechanical energy generation, absorption, and transfer amongst segments during walking. J Biomech 1980;13:845–54.
26. Helal B. Cubo-fifth metatarsal instability : a hitherto undescribed cause of pain in the outer border of the mid foot. Foot 1991;1:7–9.
27. Luciano Ade P, Lara LCR. Epidemiological study of foot and ankle injuries in recreational sports. Acta Ortop Bras 2012;20(6):339–42.
28. Ritter S, Moore M. The relationship between lateral ankle sprain and ankle tendinitis in ballet dancers. J Danc Med Sci 2008;12(1):23–31.
29. Johnson CH, Christensen JC. Biomechanics of the first ray part I: the effects of peroneus longus function: a three-dimensional kinematic study on a cadaver model. J Foot Ankle Surg 1999;38(5):313–21.
30. Rush S, Christensen JC, Johnson CH. Biomechanics of the first ray. Part II: metatarsus primus varus as a cause of hypermobility. A three-dimensional kinematic analysis in a cadaver model. J Foot Ankle Surg 2000;39(2):68–77.
31. Bierman RA, Christensen JC, Johnson CH. Biomechanics of the first ray. Part III. Consequences of Lapidus arthrodesis on peroneus longus function: a three-dimensional kinematic analysis in a cadaver model. J Foot Ankle Surg 2001; 40(3):125–31.
32. Roling BA, Christensen JC, Johnson CH. Biomechanics of the first ray. Part IV: the effect of selected medial column arthrodeses. A three-dimensional kinematic analysis in a cadaver model. J Foot Ankle Surg 2002;41(5):278–85.
33. Johnson CH, Christensen JC. Biomechanics of the first ray part V: the effect of equinus deformity. J Foot Ankle Surg 2005;44(2):114–20.
34. Roukis TS, Landsman AS. Hypermobility of the first ray: a critical review of the literature. J Foot Ankle Surg 2003;42(6):377–90.
35. Pirker W, Katzenschlager R. Gait disorders in adults and the elderly: a clinical guide. Wien Klin Wochenschr 2017;129(3–4):81–95.
36. Pérez-Soriano P, Llana-Belloch S, Morey-Klapsing G, et al. Effects of mat characteristics on plantar pressure patterns and perceived mat properties during landing in gymnastics. Sports Biomech 2010;9(4):245–57.
37. Cook T, Farrell K, Carey I, et al. Effects of restricted knee flexion and walking speed on the vertical ground reaction force during gait. J Orthop Sport Phys Ther 1997;25(4):236–44.
38. Devita P, Skelly W. Effect of landing stiffness on joint kinetics and energetics in the lower extremity. Med Sci Sports Exerc 1992;24(1):108–15.

Passive Muscular Insufficiency
The Etiology of Gastrocnemius Equinus

Jarrod Shapiro, DPM[a],*, Benjamin Kamel, DPM[b]

KEYWORDS

- Gastrocnemius equinus • Lower extremity biomechanics • Silfverskiöld
- Passive insufficiency

KEY POINTS

- The test for ankle range of motion originally described by Silfverskiöld has been incorrectly adopted for use on patients without neuromuscular diseases.
- Passive insufficiency, as in the gastrocnemius muscle, occurs in muscle/tendon units that pass across multiple joints, leading to a decrease in available range of motion of the distal joint when the proximal joint is extended.
- The unloaded, unstable foot is acted on by the normal gastrocnemius muscle complex, creating lower extremity dysfunction.

INTRODUCTION

Ankle equinus is a condition often discussed in the foot and ankle literature, and is now a term increasingly applied to various pathologic entities. Originally discussed in the orthopedic literature in relation to diseases involving muscular spasticity, most commonly cerebral palsy,[1] the concept of ankle equinus and its various treatments is now commonly applied to patients with complications related to diabetic peripheral neuropathy, pathologic flatfoot conditions, and other nonspastic lower extremity conditions.

The current opinion within the orthopedic and podiatric literature proposes that ankle equinus arises from a limitation of ankle joint dorsiflexion due to a pathologic shortening of the muscle fibers of the gastrocnemius and/or gastrocnemius-soleus muscle complex.[2] This shortening is thought to create or exacerbate pathology of the lower extremity in various ways, including increasing plantar forefoot pressures

No commercial or financial conflicts of interest and no funding sources for both authors.
[a] PMSR/RRA Podiatric Residency, Western University College of Podiatric Medicine, Chino Valley Medical Center, 309 East Second Street, Pomona, CA 91766, USA; [b] PMSR/RRA Podiatric Residency, Chino Valley Medical Center, 5451 Walnut Avenue, Chino, CA 91710, USA
* Corresponding author.
E-mail address: jshapiro@westernu.edu

leading to diabetic neuropathic ulceration[3,4] and excessive midfoot compensation in various pathologic entities.

However, an alternative evaluation of the medical literature may lead one to a different explanation of muscular ankle equinus and its role in pathology of the lower extremity. The purpose of this article is to present an alternative hypothesis of gastrocnemius equinus: diminished ankle joint dorsiflexion is a physiologic process resulting from normal functional anatomy that applies force to an already pathologic foot.

HISTORICAL BACKGROUND AND A NEW HYPOTHESIS

Early medical literature focused on ankle equinus in relation to spastic muscular disorders, especially in relation to cerebral palsy.[5] In 1923, Nils Silfverskiöld presented what became the foundation for the examination technique currently used to diagnose ankle equinus.[1] In 1971, Root and colleagues[6] defined normal ankle joint range of motion as greater than 10° dorsiflexion of the foot on the leg with the subtalar joint held in neutral position with the knee in an extended position. The investigators explained that when the foot is about to enter the toe-off phase of gait, the leg is positioned 80° to the foot, requiring 10° of dorsiflexion for appropriate gait immediately following propulsion.[5] Since then, multiple investigators proposed various definitions as well as measurement techniques discussed in detail elsewhere.[7–20]

The original literature about spastic calf muscle contracture has been extrapolated to the nonspastic patient population with the assumption that tightness of the posterior calf musculature is abnormal. It is important to note that the Silfverskiöld test, currently used for patients with nonspastic disorders, was not described for this patient population. Rather, Silfverskiöld[1] discussed this test in relation to patients with neurologic conditions and subsequent hyperactive muscle contractures.

Silfverskiöld[1] discussed the concept of "many-joints muscles," describing muscle-tendon units that pass across more than one joint. Many-joint muscles are common in the human, for example, the rectus femorus (crosses the hip and knee). The gastrocnemius muscle is also a many-joint muscle, originating on the medial condyle and lateral epicondyle of the femur and inserting on the posterior calcaneal surface, thus crossing the knee, ankle, and subtalar joints. This anatomic configuration creates the 3 joint-crossing gastrocnemius muscle.

Active and passive tension activates muscles to create forces by pulling equally on their attachments. Active tension refers to the force created in the sarcomere of activated motor units using energy stored in ATP.[21] Muscles have the unique ability to provide active forces, unlike ligaments and tendons. The shape of the active tension potential in muscle is the force-velocity relationship of muscle.[21]

When components of the muscle-tendon unit are stretched, they create a passive tension force. During a passive gastrocnemius wall stretch, the internal resistance of the Achilles tendon that prevents full range of motion is attributed to passive tension. This passive tension can be quite large and may be responsible for the muscular weakness seen in muscles following stretching.[22] Limitation of any joint range of motion is largely attributed to the passive tension created by the tendon that attaches to it. When examining passive tension on a multiarticular level, passive tension is magnified due to passive insufficiency. Elasticity also exists in the production of active muscle tension, which is likely a mixture of actin/myosin filaments, sarcomere nonuniformity, and bridge stiffness.[23–26]

The functional significance of the multijoint-crossing gastrocnemius is profound. Silfverskiöld[1] described a *transmission effect* caused by this muscular formation. When one joint in this complex moves it causes associated movement of the subsequent distal joint(s). This effect is exemplified by a runner jumping hurdles. While in mid-leap, the runner fully flexes the hip, placing the hamstring muscles on full stretch, reaching the limit of muscular length. This maximally stretched position of the hamstrings thus limits the full extension capability of the knee. Silfverskiöld[1] termed this phenomenon *passive insufficiency*. If the hip was then extended (relaxed) the hamstring muscles would now have a greater potential length, and the knee would be able to fully extend. This effect occurs throughout the body and is described by Silfverskiöld[1] as normal. In fact, it is a beneficial mechanism that increases muscular strength and decreases energy expenditure.[1]

This same transmission effect may also be applied to the gastrocnemius muscle. As noted previously, this muscle passes across multiple joints, including the knee and ankle. If one flexes the knee, the foot may be dorsiflexed on the ankle far beyond the previously stated 10° past neutral, noted as the minimum range of motion necessary for nonpathologic gait.[2,6] However, if one fully extends the knee, then the foot may be dorsiflexed on the ankle to approximately 90° and no farther (**Fig. 1**). Due to the transmission effect and passive insufficiency, the gastrocnemius muscle has reached its maximal stretch, and an apparent lack of dorsiflexion is noted. Again, this is described by Silfverskiöld[1] as being a normal physiologic process. When this same limitation occurs during gait (caused instead by an antagonist muscle actively contracting, thereby limiting joint range of motion) it is termed *active insufficiency*.

Silfverskiöld[1] described his examination technique for determining treatment of patients with spastic forms of equinus. His test is described as follows[1]:

I have tested this partly by observing the walk and partly by the following method: Passive and active dorsal flexion of the foot, with bent and with stretched knee. The degree of spasticity and passive insufficiency can be measured by the strength that is needed to produce passiv [sic] dorsal flexion of the foot with the knee bent or stretched respectively. The greater the difference in strength with bent or with stretched knee, the greater the spasticity of the gastrocnemius muscle and the passive insufficiency respectively.

Silfverskiöld[1] hypothesized that the same passive insufficiency present in the healthy human would be enhanced in patients with spastic neurologic diseases. As such, his test was simply examining the amount of spasticity rather than a pathologic contracture of the triceps surae muscle group. This test also helped him to evaluate the hypertonicity of the soleus muscle (assumed to be present if the contracture was evident with the knee both flexed and extended).

This prior research generates the foundation of a novel hypothesis: what is measured as gastrocnemius equinus is actually anatomically normal passive gastrocnemius insufficiency. Presence of "pathologic" equinus in the non-neurologically impaired patient is

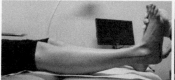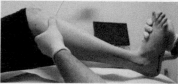

Fig. 1. The Silfverskiöld test as is commonly performed in contemporary clinical practice on this asymptomatic, healthy patient. Left image demonstrates 90° of ankle dorsiflexion with the knee extended. Right image shows the greatly improved ankle dorsiflexion with the knee flexed. Flexing the knee eliminates the transmission effect, creating greater available muscle/tendon unit length.

an erroneous diagnosis, and the Silfverskiöld[1] maneuver that is commonly performed to test for the presence of gastrocnemius versus gastrocnemius-soleus equinus is testing normal lower extremity anatomy rather than a pathologic state.

This test has been inappropriately applied to the nonspastic population in which normal passive gastrocnemius insufficiency is present. As a result, passive gastrocnemius insufficiency is incorrectly considered to be pathologic contracture. The Silfverskiöld test may be, under this new paradigm, a less essential biomechanical examination technique with decreased utility in the neurologically normal population.

RELATIONSHIP OF PASSIVE INSUFFICIENCY WITH FOOT STRUCTURE

Under optimal conditions, the foot acts through a specific timed firing of musculature, with supportive passive structures (ligaments and aponeuroses), to create a relatively "locked" foot position in late midstance.[2,27–30] The nonpathologic foot assumes this locked position, providing a mechanically stable lever arm over which the ankle dorsiflexes during midstance. The triceps surae complex fires at terminal stance, thereby plantarflexing the foot on the ankle as one unit with pedal stability maintained.

To summarize, the normal action of the triceps surae is predicated on a "preloaded" foot, which has an appropriately supinated subtalar position, creating a stable foot position in which to plantarflex during the push-off period of the stance phase of gait.

The foot may become preloaded through a variety of proposed mechanisms, including, but likely not limited to the following:

- Subtalar supination leading to a "locked" midtarsal position.[2,31,32]
- Close packed position of the calcaneocuboid joint leading to an advantageous position of the peroneus longus and plantarflexion of the first metatarsal with subsequent retrograde plantarflexion of the medial column (close packed medial column position) and stable medial longitudinal arch.[28,33]
- Tibialis posterior muscle concentric action on the midtarsal and subtalar joints.[2]
- The windlass mechanism provides passive stability at terminal stance and toe off.[34]
- Bony architecture, with the medial arch keystone effect, provides passive medial longitudinal arch stability.[34,35]

If these preloading mechanisms fail, then the foot remains in a loose "unloaded" position with loss of mechanical stability. When normal ankle dorsiflexion occurs at midstance (in the presence of normal anatomic passive gastrocnemius insufficiency) the foot is unprepared to accept the forces of the triceps surae proximally and ground reactive forces plantarly. The subtalar joint will increasingly pronate as compensation leading to the typical flatfoot appearance. At toe off, when the ankle is plantarflexing and triceps surae actively firing, the unstable condition is further worsened with midfoot dorsiflexion as compensation for the lack of ankle dorsiflexion.

Various mechanisms have been proposed to explain the causes of an unstable foot, such as the subtalar joint neutral theory proposed by Root and colleagues[2] and rotational equilibrium theory of Kirby.[36] Passive gastrocnemius insufficiency may be incorporated into this system as well. In the pathologic foot, if the tibialis posterior and peroneus longus contract too late or inefficiently due to pathologic events described previously, then unstable structures are overpowered by an otherwise anatomically normal triceps surae complex.

The phenomenon of "early heel off" in the pathologically pronated foot also may be explained through the lens of passive insufficiency. Early heel off is seen clinically during the midstance phase of gait and may occur due to a normal passive gastrocnemius insufficiency acting on a pathologically non-preloaded foot that dorsiflexes at the mid-foot (**Fig. 2**, right). The same is true for early heel off in the pes cavus type foot except the foot is appropriately preloaded and the entire foot elevates off the ground early as a result of passive gastrocnemius insufficiency (see **Fig. 2**, left).

RELATIONSHIP OF CURRENT RESEARCH TO PASSIVE INSUFFICIENCY

All current research literature has assumed pathologic gastrocnemius equinus, rather than normal passive insufficiency. This factor may be part of the explanation for the controversy behind the variable measuring techniques as well as the definition of ankle equinus itself.[14–19]

Hill[37] prospectively examined 176 of 209 consecutive new patients presenting to a foot and ankle clinic over a 6-week period. Of the 176 patients with a biomechanically related complaint, 96.5% also had equinus defined as less than 3° ankle joint dorsi-flexion using a tractograph. Hill[37] concluded the high incidence of equinus reflected an "acquired deformity." It is difficult to extrapolate these numbers to the healthy pop-ulation because gathering data from a clinic leads to selection bias in favor of symp-tomatic patients. However, despite this, the high incidence may be explained by the normal presence of passive gastrocnemius insufficiency rather than an acquired deformity.

Saxena and Kim[38] in 2003 looked at the prevalence of ankle equinus in a healthy adolescent athlete population. Using a hand-held goniometer with patients supine and foot in neutral position, they examined 40 healthy high school athletes, measuring ankle joint dorsiflexion with the knee both extended and flexed. Mean ankle dorsiflexion in this asymptomatic young, athletic population was found to be zero degrees with the knee extended and 5° with the knee flexed. The inves-tigators explained their method of measurement and small cohort as limiting factors with increased potential for variability. They hypothesized, "Adolescent ath-letes have a component of gastrocnemius equinus." These findings in a young, healthy, asymptomatic population may be more adequately explained by the pres-ence of anatomic passive gastrocnemius insufficiency rather than a pathologic process.

DiGiovanni and colleagues[32] compared ankle joint range of motion in 2 groups of patients. Group 1 consisted of 34 patients with metatarsalgia and related forefoot

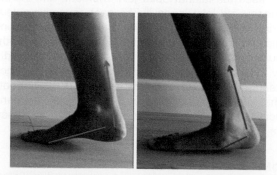

Fig. 2. In the left image, the Achilles transmits its force to an intact medial longitudinal arch via a long lever arm with normal heel elevation. In the right image, a pathologic medial lon-gitudinal arch dorsiflexes during push off, creating a short lever arm on which the Achilles tendon may act. In both cases, the gastrocnemius-soleus complex is normal but acting on a pathologic foot in the right image.

and midfoot symptoms, whereas the control group consisted of 34 patients without foot or ankle pain. These investigators measured ankle range of motion using an equinometer (goniometer linked to a pressure sensor to standardize the amount of pressure when dorsiflexing the foot with computerized angle determination). They found a significant difference in the amount of ankle dorsiflexion between groups. However, in both groups, a difference was noted in the amount of ankle dorsiflexion with the knee extended versus flexed. These results may, again, be explained by gastrocnemius passive insufficiency. However, potential confounding issues are demonstrated with this study due to methodological limitations. The experimental and control groups were heterogeneous. Five patients in the experimental group had diabetes, whereas none in the control group did. This may have led to a selection bias toward decreased ankle range of motion because diabetic individuals have been shown to have glycosylation of tendons.[39,40] Seven patients in the experimental group were smokers versus 3 in the control group. It is unknown what specific effect smoking has on tendon length and function, although it is considered detrimental to appropriate tendon function.[41] In addition, 5 members of the control group had ligamentous laxity whereas only 1 in the experimental group did, pointing again to heterogeneity of sample groups. Based on the study's limitations, the investigators' conclusions may be inaccurate.

Lavery and colleagues[3] examined 1666 diabetic patients in a prospective observational cohort study. They found an ankle equinus (defined as <0° dorsiflexion at the ankle) prevalence of 10.3% in this cohort, which is significantly lower than prior studies. This may be because of their definition of equinus, which would have underestimated limitation of ankle range of motion. In addition, the method of examination was not stated, making this study difficult to compare with prior research.

Similarly, Frykberg and colleagues[42] in 2012, while prospectively comparing equinus in 43 diabetic versus 59 nondiabetic patients found a 24.5% prevalence (odds ratio 3.3). These researchers used a biplane goniometer to measure ankle joint range of motion with a definition identical to Lavery and colleagues.[3] Similarly, the definition of equinus may have affected the observed prevalence.

Surgical biomechanical research additionally lends support to this concept. In 2009, Arangio and Salathe[43] compared the force of a 10-mm medial displacement calcaneal osteotomy on the medial column ligaments of an experimental cadaver flatfoot with intact foot as a control. The calcaneal osteotomy decreased first metatarsal force, decreased the talonavicular joint moment, and increased fifth metatarsal and calcaneocuboid joint loads.[43] The gastrocnemius-soleus complex was not modified during the study and had no effect on the outcome. Creating an abnormally functioning medial column was the primary factor in this experimental model. Similar outcomes were found with the use of subtalar arthroeiresis[44] and Evans osteotomy.[45] Nyska and colleagues[46] further found that increasing the pull of the Achilles tendon in a cadaver model increased the flatfoot deformity, but only in the feet that were made unstable by sectioning the ligaments of the medial column. An artificially tightened Achilles tendon only had an effect on the experimentally unstable foot.

FUTURE DIRECTIONS

This model calls into question the modern concept of muscular ankle equinus. Understanding correct physiologic function is a prerequisite to advancing medical science and patient care, and future research may demonstrate modifications to nonsurgical and surgical methodology.

Contemporary applications of this new hypothesis may be considered in both the nonsurgical and surgical realms. For example, during reconstructive surgery for pathologic pronatory conditions, it is common to perform either a tendoachilles lengthening or gastrocnemius recession with the intent to reduce what was previously considered a pathologic equinus. However, with this alternative model, the goal of flatfoot surgery would be to first create a stable foot with an improved ability to preload, allowing the normal gastrocnemius muscle to function appropriately. One purpose of the medial displacement calcaneal osteotomy is to medialize the pull of the tendoachilles (in addition to placing the calcaneal bisection in line with the tibia). If the triceps surae insertion were placed medial to the subtalar joint axis (rather than lateral to it) the gastrocnemius muscle would be altered from a subtalar joint pronator to supinator. In this case, performing a gastrocnemius recession or tendoachilles lengthening procedure would be contraindicated in flatfoot surgery. A normal triceps surae redirected to an improved anatomic location would be a more effective lever than an artificially lengthened one.

Similarly, foot orthosis therapy may benefit from a more accurate anatomic model. A current application of this concept may be to incorporate a heel lift into the orthosis shell to limit passive insufficiency. This method is supported by a study by Johanson and colleagues,[16] who found increased ankle dorsiflexion and increased time to heel off in patients with less than 5° ankle dorsiflexion after placement of a 6-mm or 9-mm heel lift.

A review of the literature reveals that it has never been asked how a pathologic contracture of the gastrocnemius muscle can be so prevalent in the human population. Despite the apparent high prevalence of gastrocnemius equinus, most researchers have assumed this is pathologic. In reality it is not the "pathologic" contracture of this muscle that creates foot dysfunction but rather the normal passive insufficiency created by the gastrocnemius being a multijoint muscle. Further research is necessary to confirm this hypothesis before it is accepted into common clinical practice.

REFERENCES

1. Silfverskiöld N. Reduction of the uncrossed two-joints muscles of the leg to one-joint muscles in spastic conditions. Acta Chir Scand 1924;56:315.
2. Root M, Orien W, Weed J. Normal and abnormal function of the foot: clinical biomechanics volume II. Los Angeles (CA): Clinical Biomechanics Corporation; 1977.
3. Lavery L, Armstrong D, Boulton A. Ankle equinus deformity and its relationship to high plantar pressure in a large population with diabetes mellitus. J Am Podiatr Med Assoc 2002;92:479.
4. Mueller M, Sinacore D, Hastings M, et al. Effect of Achilles tendon lengthening on neuropathic plantar ulcers: a randomized clinical trial. J Bone Joint Surg 2003; 85-A:1436.
5. Hibbs R. Muscle bound feet. New York Med J 1914;17C:797.
6. Root M, Orien W, Weed J. Biomechanical examination of the foot, Volume 1. Los Angeles (CA): Clinical Biomechanics Corporation; 1971.
7. Hillstrom H, Perlberg G, Siegler S, et al. Objective identification of ankle equinus deformity and resulting contracture. J Am Podiatr Med Assoc 1991;81:519.
8. DiGiovanni CW, Holt S, Czerniecki JM, et al. Can the presence of equinus contracture be determined by physical exam alone? J Rehabil Res Dev 2001; 38:335.

9. Charles J, Scutter SD, Buckley J. Static ankle joint equinus: toward a standard definition and diagnosis. J Am Podiatr Med Assoc 2010;100:195.
10. Young R, Nix S, Wholohan A, et al. Interventions for increasing ankle joint dorsiflexion: a systematic review and meta-analysis. J Foot Ankle Res 2013;6(1):46.
11. Charles J, Scutter SD, Buckley J. Static ankle joint equinus: toward a standard definition and diagnosis. J Am Podiatr Med Assoc 2012;100(3):195–203.
12. Wren TA, Do KP, Kay RM. Gastrocnemius and soleus lengths in cerebral palsy equinus gait–differences between children with and without static contracture and effects of gastrocnemius recession. J Biomech 2004;37(9):1321–7.
13. Downey MS, Schwartz JM. Ankle equinus. In: Southerland JT, editor. McGlamry's comprehensive textbook of foot and ankle surgery. Philadelphia: Wolters Kluwer Health/Lippincott Williams & Wilkins; 2013. p. 541–84.
14. Gatt A, Chockalingam N. Validity and reliability of a new ankle dorsiflexion measurement device. Prosthet Orthot Int 2013;37(4):289–97.
15. Martin RL, Mcpoil TG. Reliability of ankle goniometric measurements: a literature review. J Am Podiatr Med Assoc 2005;95(6):564–72.
16. Johanson MA, Dearment A, Hines K, et al. The effect of subtalar joint position on dorsiflexion of the ankle/rearfoot versus midfoot/forefoot during gastrocnemius stretching. Foot Ankle Int 2014;35(1):63–70.
17. O'Shea S, Grafton K. The intra and inter-rater reliability of a modified weight-bearing lunge measure of ankle dorsiflexion. Man Ther 2013;18(3):264–8.
18. Bennell KL, Talbot RC, Wajswelner H, et al. Intra-rater and inter-rater reliability of a weight-bearing lunge measure of ankle dorsiflexion. Aust J Physiother 1998; 44(3):175–80.
19. Munteanu SE, Strawhorn AB, Landorf KB, et al. A weightbearing technique for the measurement of ankle joint dorsiflexion with the knee extended is reliable. J Sci Med Sport 2009;12(1):54–9.
20. Perry J. Ankle foot complex: gait analysis: normal and pathology function. Thorofare (NJ): SLACK, Inc; 1992. p. 51–88.
21. Knudson D. Fundamentals of biomechanics. 2nd edition. New York: Springer; 2007. p. 51–66.
22. Knudson D, Magnusson P, McHugh M. Current issues in flexibility fitness. Pres Counc Phys Fit Sports Res Dig 2000;3(9):1–8.
23. Huijing PA, Baan GC. Extramuscular myofascial force transmission within the rat anterior tibial compartment: proximo-distal differences in muscle force. Acta Physiol Scand 2001;173:1–15.
24. Huijing PA, Baan GC. Myofascial force transmission causes interaction between adjacent muscles and connective tissue: effects of blunt dissection and compartmental fasciotomy on length force characteristics of rat extensor digitorum longus muscle. Arch Physiol Biochem 2001;109:97–109.
25. Huijing PA, Baan GC. Myofascial force transmission: muscle relative position and length determine agonist and synergist muscle force. J Appl Physiol (1985) 2003; 94:1092–107.
26. Huijing PA, Baan GC, Rebel G. Non myo-tendinous force transmission in rat extensor digitorum longus muscle. J Exp Biol 1998;201:682–91.
27. Roling B, Christensen J, Johnson C. Biomechanics of the first ray part IV. The effect of selected medial column arthrodeses: a three-dimensional kinematic study on a cadaver model. J Foot Ankle Surg 2002;41(5):278–85.
28. Johnson C, Christensen J. Biomechanics of the first ray part 1. The effects of peroneus longus function: a three-dimensional kinematic study on a cadaver model. J Foot Ankle Surg 1999;38(5):313–21.

29. Bojsen-Moller F. Calcaneocuboid joint and stability of the longitudinal arch of the foot at high and low gear push off. J Anat 1979;129(1):165–76.
30. Hicks JH. Chapter 7: the three weight-bearing mechanisms of the foot. In: Evan FG, editor. Biomechanical studies of the musculoskeletal system. Springfield (IL): Charles C. Thomas; 1961.
31. Elftman H. The transverse tarsal joint and its control. Clin Orthop 1960;16:41–6.
32. DiGiovanni CW, Kuo R, Tejwani N, et al. Isolated gastrocnemius tightness. J Bone Joint Surg Am 2002;84(6):962–70.
33. Perez HR, Reber LK, Christensen JC. The effect of frontal plane position on first ray motion: forefoot locking mechanism. Foot Ankle Int 2008;29(1):72–6.
34. Hicks JH. The mechanics of the foot. J Anat 1953;87(4):345–57.
35. Ouzounian T, Shereff M. In vitro determination of midfoot motion. Foot Ankle 1989; 10(3):140–6.
36. Kirby K. Subtalar joint axis location and rotational equilibrium theory of foot function. J Am Podiatr Med Assoc 2001;91:465.
37. Hill R. Ankle equinus: prevalence and linkage to common foot pathology. J Am Podiatr Med Assoc 1995;85:295.
38. Saxena A, Kim W. Ankle dorsiflexion in adolescent athletes. J Am Podiatr Med Assoc 2003;93:312.
39. Giacomozzi C, D'ambrogi E, Uccioli L, et al. Does the thickening of Achilles tendon and plantar fascia contribute to the alteration of diabetic foot loading? Clin Biomech 2005;20:532.
40. Reddy G. Cross-linking in collagen by nonenzymatic glycation increases the matrix stiffness in rabbit achilles tendon. Exp Diabesity Res 2004;5:143.
41. Lee J, Patel R, Biermann J, et al. Musculoskeletal effects of smoking. JBJS 2013; 95-A:850.
42. Frykberg R, Bowen J, Hall J, et al. Prevalence of equinus in diabetic versus nondiabetic patients. J Am Podiatr Med Assoc 2012;102:84.
43. Arangio G, Salathe E. A biomechanical analysis of posterior tibial tendon dysfunction, medial displacement calcaneal osteotomy and flexor digitorum longus transfer in adult acquired flatfoot. Clin Biomech 2009;24:385–90.
44. Arangio G, Reinert KL, Salathe EP, et al. A biomechanical model of the effect of subtalar arthroereisis on the adult flexible flat foot. Clin Biomech 2004;19:847–52.
45. Arangio G, Chopra V, Voloshin A, et al. A biomechanical analysis of the effect of lateral column lengthening calcaneal osteotomy of flatfoot. Clin Biomech 2007;22: 472–7.
46. Nyska M, Parks BG, Chu IT, et al. The contribution of the medial calcaneal osteotomy to the correction of flatfoot deformities. Foot Ankle Int 2001;22(4):278–82.

Biomechanics and Orthotic Treatment of the Adult Acquired Flatfoot

Douglas Richie, DPM*

KEYWORDS

• Adult acquired flatfoot • PTTD • Posterior tibial tendon • AFO devices

KEY POINTS

• The adult acquired flatfoot deformity arises from attenuation and functional rupture of the posterior tibial tendon and the combined rupture of the spring ligament complex and the deltoid ligament complex.

• This deformity is characterized by hindfoot eversion, collapse of the medial longitudinal arch, and forefoot abduction.

• The pivotal joint in adult acquired flatfoot is the talonavicular joint, destabilized by rupture of the spring ligament complex.

INTRODUCTION

The adult acquired flatfoot (AAF), secondary to posterior tibial tendon dysfunction (PTTD) poses a significant challenge to not only the patient, but also the treating clinician. Despite there being more than 350 articles published in the medical literature on the subject of PTTD since 1990, there remains a lack of universal agreement about the etiology and preferred treatment of the condition.[1] Not withstanding, careful review of recent studies can provide insight into the pathomechanics of AAF to help direct a treatment program using orthotic intervention.

TERMINOLOGY

In 2017, Ross and colleagues evaluated the evolution of the terms "posterior tibial tendon dysfunction" and "adult acquired flatfoot deformity."[1] After systematic

Disclosure: Dr D. Richie is the owner of Richie Technologies Inc, which markets ankle-foot orthoses.
Applied Biomechanics, California School of Podiatric Medicine, Samuel Merritt University, Oakland, CA, USA
* 550 Pacific Coast Highway, Suite 209, Seal Beach, CA 90740.
E-mail address: drichiejr@aol.com

Table 1
Johnson and Strom classification of PTTD

	Stage 1	Stage 2	Stage 3	Stage 4
Posterior tibial tendon	Tenosynovitis, degeneration, or both	Elongation and degeneration	Elongation and degeneration	Elongation and degeneration
Deformity	Absent	Flexible, reducible pes planovalgus deformity with hindfoot held in equines	Fixed, irreducible pes planovalgus deformity	Fixed, irreducible pes planovalgus deformity
Pain	Medial	Medial, lateral or both	Medial, lateral or both	Medial, lateral or both
Single limb heel-risc	Mild weakness; hindfool inverts normally	Marked weakness; no or weak inversion of hindfoot	Unable to perform test; no inversion of hindfoot	Unable to perform test; no inversion of hindfoot
Too many toes sign	Negative	Positive	Positive	Positive
Valgus deformity and arthritis of ankle	No	No	No	Yes

review of the medical literature, Ross and colleagues recognized that the two terms could actually describe two different clinical conditions or pathologies. PTTD is limiting as it describes a condition that depends on tendon function, while overlooking the role of ligamentous failure.[2,3] PTTD can occur in early stages without significant foot deformity.[4] The most popular classification system for PTTD relies solely on the integrity of the posterior tibial tendon (**Table 1**). AAF describes a foot deformity that can be the result of tendon rupture and/or ligament rupture as well as other conditions such as Charcot arthropathy, rheumatoid arthritis, or neurologic disorder.[1,5–7] In this article, the AAF is defined as a symptomatic, progressive deformity of the foot caused by a loss of dynamic, and static supportive structures of the medial longitudinal arch.[8]

CLINICAL PRESENTATION

The typical patient with AAF is a middle-aged to elderly woman presenting with pain and swelling along the medial ankle.[9] Frequently, the patient will have noticed a visible collapse of the medial longitudinal arch.[10] The symptoms are almost always unilateral, while the patient has been aware of being flatfooted all of their life.[11–13]

Patients with AAF have been identified to have significant comorbidities. Holmes and Mann[14] were among the first to study risk factors associated with rupture of the posterior tibial tendon in patients they treated over an 8-year period at their clinics. Of the 67 patients, 51 were women, thus making up 76% of the patient pool. There was a strong correlation with obesity ($P = .005$) followed by hypertension ($P = .025$). Fifty-two percent of the patients had either diabetes, hypertension, or obesity. With advanced age, obesity, and other risk factors, surgical intervention for patients with AAF are always carefully considered only after conservative treatment has failed.[15,16]

ANATOMY

The tibialis posterior (TP) originates in the proximal portion of the lower leg from the tibia, the fibula, and the interosseous membrane. Morimoto[17] demonstrated that the fibular side of this origin is strongest, improving the lever arm for transverse and frontal plane control of the foot and ankle.

The TP is a multipennate muscle with short fibers designed for short excursion and more powerful contraction. Shorter muscle fiber length equates to increased strength. Silver and associates[18] evaluated strength of the lower extremity musculature by measuring the volume of each muscle and then dividing by muscle fiber length. The soleus is the strongest muscle crossing the ankle joint accounting for 30% of the strength of the lower leg musculature and the gastrocnemius provides 19.2% of overall strength. In comparison the TP provides only 6.4% of the strength of the lower extremity musculature and the flexor digitorum longus (FDL) provides 1.8%.

The tendon of the TP, also know as the posterior tibial tendon, originates at the myotendon junction located above the medial malleolus. There are 6 sections of the posterior tibial tendon: myotendon transition, proximal retinaculum, retromalleolar, inframalleolar, distal retinaculum, and insertion.[19] The TP tendon changes direction at the distal margin of the medial malleolus and takes on a distinct histologic appearance owing to the physical forces that result from the bony pulley at this location. In this retromalleolar region is a section of fibrocartilage on the anterior surface of the TP tendon, which provides a gliding surface that protects against compression and shear stress.[20,21] This fibrocartilage has been speculated to also interrupt the normal blood flow to the PT tendon.[22] Several studies have identified a so-called hypovascular zone of the PT tendon beginning in the retromalleolar region and extending 1.4 cm distal to the tip of the medial malleolus.[23,24] However, Prado and colleagues[25] conducted their own study of perfusion of the PT tendon and concluded there was no zone of hypovascularity, and the vulnerability for rupture of this tendon in the retromalleolar region can be attributed to mechanical stresses that arise from a flatfoot deformity.

There are 3 main components of the insertion of the TP tendon. It is important for every clinician to appreciate these components and multiple insertions of this tendon and how they affect overall foot function and stability. The anterior component is the largest and inserts on the tuberosity of the navicular as well as the first (medial) cuneiform.[19] The middle component is most important functionally because it inserts on the second and third cuneiforms as well as the cuboid. Other slips of the middle component insert on the base of metatarsals second, third, fourth, and sometimes the fifth metatarsals.[19] The middle component also gives attachment to the medial limb of origin of the flexor hallucis brevis muscle. Finally, the third component is a recurrent slip of the TP tendon, which inserts on the anterior aspect of the sustentaculum tali.

The spring ligament complex is probably the most important anatomic structure of the AAF because it is commonly ruptured in this condition and the biomechanical consequences are severe.[26,27] The first detailed description of an actual complex of ligaments collectively termed the spring ligament was published by Davis and colleagues[28] in 1996. Since that time, many detailed anatomic studies have been published, which verify that multiple ligaments as well as a continuous capsule make up both the spring ligament and the deltoid ligament complexes.[29–36] These studies verify the following findings regarding the static support of the medial ankle and medial longitudinal arch:

1. The deltoid and spring ligaments are part of one continuous capsule extending from the distal tibia to the calcaneus and the navicular.

2. There are 4 components of the medial collateral ligament complex: The tibiocalcanealnavicular (TCN), superficial posterior tibiotalar, deep posterior tibiotalar, and deep anterior tibiotalar ligaments.
3. The spring ligament complex is composed of the superomedial calcaneonavicular and the inferoplantar ligaments.
4. The spring ligament actually has its origin proximally on the distal tibia via the TCN ligament, which has 3 branches: the tibionavicular, tibiospring, and tibiocalcaneal.
5. The TCN, via the superomedial calcaneonavicular ligament articulates with the plantar and medial aspect of the head of the talus via a section of cartilaginous tissue. This ligament restrains plantar-medial migration of the head of the talus
6. The TCN, via the tibiocalcaneal ligament, restrains frontal plane eversion of the subtalar joint.
7. The deep posterior tibiotalar ligament is the strongest stabilizer of the talocrural joint.

WHAT IS THE FUNCTION OF THE TIBIALIS POSTERIOR?

Traditionally, the TP has been called the "strongest invertor of the foot."[10,11,37,38] This belief has been based on simple observation of the location of the proximal portion of the TP tendon relative to the head and neck of the talus, that is, the subtalar joint.[12] Viewing the location of the TP tendon in the transverse plane, relative to the axis of the subtalar joint, this tendon would be most medially located and would therefore have the longest lever arm for inversion compared with all other tendons. This notion was supported by Hintermann and colleagues[39] in an in vitro cadaver study. In this study, the TP tendon was given a value of 1.0 inversion moment arm, whereas the FDL scored 0.75 and the tibialis anterior scored 0.59.

McCullough and colleagues[40] noted some deficiencies in the Hintermann study as well as other previous published works on the subject of muscle moment arms in the lower extremity. Using a simulator with more modern methods of measuring tendon moment arms, McCullough and colleagues determined that the longest, most effective moment arm for foot inversion is provided by the tibialis anterior (16 mm), which was 30% longer than the TP (10 mm). The most effective moment arm provided by the TP is in the transverse plane(adduction/abduction) where the moment arm measures 21.4 mm.

If we combine the knowledge of moment arm length with previous studies of muscle strength, a calculation of overall torque or joint moment can be made.[40–42] For inversion the TP is capable of generating 7.5 N-meters (Nm) of torque and the tibialis anterior can generate 5.8 Nm. For adduction, the TP generates 15.7 Nm and the FDL generates 3.8 Nm.

Clearly, the torque-producing activity of the TP is twice as great in the transverse plane as the frontal plane. If lost, the TP can be supported in the direction of inversion by another muscle with similar torque producing capacity: the tibialis anterior. However, in the transverse plane, supplemental adduction torque produced by the FDL achieves only one-fourth the power of the TP. This finding explains why the AAF deformity is most dominant in the transverse plane rather than the frontal plane.[8]

PATHOMECHANICS OF THE ADULT ACQUIRED FLATFOOT

The true pathomechanics of the AAF remains a topic of debate. Historically, the disorder has been attributed to a loss of function of the TP muscle or tendon.[2,9,10,43] The classification system most commonly used in published studies of AAF is based solely on function of the posterior tibial tendon.[3] Yet, many studies subsequent to the early reports demonstrated that the AAF deformity does not occur with isolated rupture of the posterior tibial tendon.[11,26,44,45] In cadaveric studies, multiple ligaments must be severed before visible change of alignment occurs as seen in stage 2 AAF deformity[46–49] (**Fig. 1**). Of these ligaments, the spring ligament complex seems to be most critical.

In a landmark study, Jennings and Christensen[50] sectioned the spring ligament in 5 cadaveric specimens subjected to axial load while also loading the posterior tibial tendon. When the spring ligament was sectioned, a significant change of alignment associated with flatfoot deformity occurred, for which the posterior tibial tendon was unable to compensate. These findings were further validated in a more recent study using finite analysis computer modeling to measure stress in key soft tissue structures in stage 2 AAF deformity.[51] The plantar aponeurosis and the spring ligament were the 2 primary structures to maintain integrity of the medial longitudinal arch, and the TP tendon played a secondary role. Furthermore, the plantar aponeurosis has a primary role to prevent arch elongation. The spring ligament was found to have a primary function of controlling motion at the talonavicular and subtalar joints.

What is almost universally agreed upon is that PTTD begins with a preexisting flatfoot deformity.[2,3,10–12] From this observation, there was early speculation that the flatfoot deformity places increased mechanical load on the TP muscle and tendon, without any scientific validation.[3,52] Subsequent to these early reports, interesting insight into muscle function in patients with pes planus as well as mechanical loads on the TP tendon has been gained from in vitro and in vivo studies.

Murley and colleagues[53] studied electromyography muscle activity in 30 adults with flat arched feet and compared them with 30 adults with normal arched feet during walking. During the contact phase of gait, the flat arched group demonstrated increased activity of the tibialis anterior and decreased activity of the peroneus longus muscles. During midstance and propulsion, patients with flat arches exhibited increased activity of the TP and decreased activity of the peroneus longus in comparison with those patients with normal arched feet. Therefore, a flatfoot posture creates more demand on the foot invertors and has decreased the demand on the evertors

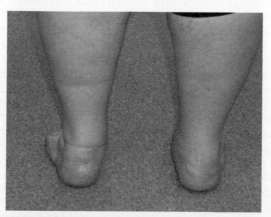

Fig. 1. Stage 2 AAF demonstrated by asymmetrical deformity on left side, hindfoot valgus and forefoot abduction, that is, the too many toes sign.

during gait. Two other electromyography studies have found similar findings of increased activity of the tibialis anterior and TP in patients with pes planus and pronated foot posture.[54,55]

At the level of the TP tendon, interesting insight has been gained from studies of friction force at the level of the medial malleolus and bony pulley, which develops at the 90° turn of this tendon, moving from the leg into the foot.

This location has already been identified to be a site of increased gliding motion, formation of adaptive cartilage, and resultant decreased vascularity.[20–24] Any area of tendon exposed to increased friction in a gliding zone could be susceptible to cumulative trauma and tendon degeneration.[56,57] Uchiyama and colleagues[58] studied the gliding resistance of the posterior tibial tendon at various positions of the foot. Dorsiflexion of the ankle in the cadaveric specimens increased gliding resistance, whereas plantarflexion decreased gliding resistance. Creation of a flatfoot deformity caused a 30% increased gliding resistance of the posterior tibial tendon. This increased gliding resistance in a preexisting flatfoot model was speculated to be a precursor to mechanical overload, and eventual structural failure of the posterior tibial tendon.

A subsequent study by Arai and colleagues[59] validated increased friction work by the posterior tibial tendon in a flatfoot deformity, particularly in the transverse and frontal planes. Also, this study showed increased friction of the TP tendon with increased loading of the foot, suggesting that body mass and obesity are contributing factors. Finally, a study by Fujii and colleagues[60] determined that the FDL and flexor hallucis longus do not increase gliding resistance in a simulated flatfoot condition.

It seems that the unique anatomic location of the TP tendon in the malleolar groove provides the setting for increased friction of this tendon, particularly when the foot is moved in the direction of abduction and eversion.

Degeneration, attenuation, and eventual rupture of the TP tendon are important parts of the pathomechanics of the AAF, but does not explain the deformity. It seems that rupture of the spring ligament complex is the key step in the AAF and this is thought to occur in early stage 2, when asymmetrical deformity of the affected foot is visible clinically.[26,44] However, in vitro cadaver studies do not show immediate collapse of the arch with severing of the spring ligament. Only with cyclical loading and attenuation of other ligaments will visible collapse of the arch occur.[27,61,62]

Deland and colleagues[26] performed an MRI evaluation of 31 patients with documented evidence of degeneration or tear of the TP tendon. The superomedial portion of the spring ligament was attenuated or torn in 87% of the patients. The talocalcaneal interosseous ligament was affected in 48% of the patients. Although signal change in the plantar fascia was present in 26% of the patients, no partial or complete tears were noted. Balen and Helms[63] had similar findings of spring ligament injury in their MRI study, and also did not find significant tears of the plantar fascia in patients with AAF. Although these studies show signal changes associated with fasciitis from overload, frank rupture of the plantar aponeurosis is not seen in patients with AAF.

After rupture of the spring ligament, it is postulated that the superficial deltoid ligament attenuates and ruptures. Specifically, Ormsby and associates[64] identified in MRI studies that the talonavicular component of the superficial deltoid ligament ruptures after the spring ligament in AAF. The tibiocalcaneal component of the superficial deltoid ligament also ruptures in AAF, accounting for unrestrained eversion of the calcaneus. This shifts the insertion of the Achilles tendon lateral to the subtalar joint axis, adding further valgus moment to the hindfoot. As the medial arch collapses, the calcaneus plantarflexes, leading to contracture of the Achilles tendon.[65,66] This contracture has always been assumed to be a secondary or acquired finding rather than a primary causative factor in AAF deformity.[4,10,12]

What causes the initial rupture of the spring ligament leading to AAF remains unknown. One long-held theory is that a congenital flatfoot deformity is associated with subtalar joint pronation that unlocks the midtarsal joint.[3,10,12] Increased sagittal plane motion across the midfoot joints with subtalar joint pronation has been verified in multiple studies.[67] This increased flexibility across the midfoot is thought to place repetitive load on the static supportive structures of the medial arch, specifically the spring ligament.[68,69] A newer theory is based on an understanding of the intimate relationship between the posterior tibial tendon and the spring ligament complex.[70] This complex forms the floor of the synovial sheath of the TP tendon.[28,36] A tear of this tendon could extend into the spring ligament owing to the blending of the 2 structures just proximal to the navicular. Or, the loss of physical reinforcement of the spring ligament, which would occur with TP tendon rupture, would possibly explain why this ligament would also be at risk for subsequent rupture.

GAIT STUDIES OF ADULT ACQUIRED FLATFOOT

Rattanaprasert and coworkers[71] were the first to study gait in a PTTD patient using a 3-dimensional multisegment foot model. The study subject was not a typical AAF patient because she was 35 years of age and had suffered a traumatic rupture of the TP tendon at age 6. Compared with a group of 10 healthy patients, the TP rupture patient showed excessive dorsiflexion of the forefoot on the rearfoot at 70% of the stance phase of gait, just before heel rise. This finding indicated significant loss of stiffness of the medial arch of the foot owing to TP rupture. Also, the patient exhibited excessive abduction of the forefoot at midstance and lack of adduction after heel rise.

Tome and colleagues[72] used a multisegment foot model with a marker on the navicular to measure medial longitudinal arch angle in 12 patients with PTTD compared with 10 healthy controls. In the patients with PTTD, greater forefoot abduction was measured from loading response through terminal stance compared with controls. The medial longitudinal arch angle was significantly lower through preswing in the patients with PTTD. The investigators concluded that after rupture of the TP tendon, other muscles of the lower leg are unable to compensate and provide stability to the foot. The loss of alignment of the arch suggests that an osseous locking mechanism does not exist in the foot, and arch integrity depends on ligaments, specifically the plantar aponeurosis and the spring ligament. In their conclusion, the authors stated, "The data from the current study suggest the choice of orthoses or brace should focus on the ability of the device to control rearfoot eversion, MLA angle, and forefoot abduction across the entire stance period."[72]

Ringleb and colleagues[73] studied the kinematics, plantar foot pressures, and electromyography activity in 5 patients with PTTD. As with previous studies, increased forefoot dorsiflexion across the midfoot joints was observed in the patients with PTTD. In addition, a varus motion of the forefoot during heel rise was measured in these patients, whereas healthy controls showed forefoot pronation during this phase, indicating healthy function of the first ray and engagement of the windlass mechanism. In this study, patients with PTTD exhibited greater activity of the peroneus longus, perhaps a compensation attempting to evert the forefoot and plantarflex the first ray. Also, increased activity of the gastrocnemius was measured in the PTTD group, suggesting excessive work to plantarflex the ankle with an unstable midfoot.

Houck and colleagues[74] used a multisegment foot model to evaluate rearfoot motion and midfoot motion as well as first metatarsal motion in 30 patients with PTTD compared with 15 healthy controls. The patient group demonstrated greater hindfoot eversion, greater plantarflexion of the rearfoot on the forefoot, and greater first metatarsal dorsiflexion through the stance phase of gait. Lowering of the medial longitudinal arch was due largely to first metatarsal dorsiflexion. The plantarflexed attitude of the rearfoot was speculated to shorten the Achilles tendon and cause weakness for push off. This may explain why patients with PTTD demonstrate a delayed heel off.[75] However, instability and increased flexibility of the medial arch and midfoot joints would also compromise the ability of the triceps to transfer plantarflexion moment to the forefoot during terminal stance.

Neville and colleagues[76] studied plantar-loading patterns in patients with PTTD. A decrease in total loading of the forefoot during terminal stance in the patient group indicated loss of stability of the arch for push off. Furthermore, there was a loss of lateral forefoot loading, which would normally occur with hindfoot inversion. A shift of loading toward the midfoot and heel was similar to what is seen in patients with rupture of the Achilles tendon. With the loss of arch and midfoot stability, the Achilles tendon seems to be ineffective in transferring load to the forefoot in patients with PTTD. This can be demonstrated when patients with stage 2 deformity are unable to perform a single foot heel rise (**Fig. 2**). In a follow-up study, this same research group determined that the loss of normal loading of the forefoot during terminal stance in PTTD is not due to muscle weakness, but rather due to loss of ligament stability across the midfoot joints.[77]

Van de Velde and colleagues[78] were the first to compare patient stage 2 and stage 3 AAF kinematic variables and measure coupling between key segments of the foot and leg. As expected, the more rigid stage 3 deformity was associated with less motion of the rearfoot and the medial arch compared with stage 2. Both groups demonstrated decreased walking speed and delayed heel lift compared with healthy controls. Verifying previous studies, AAF is associated with reduced hindfoot inversion and forefoot

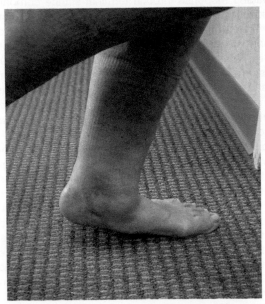

Fig. 2. Unstable midfoot during single foot heel rise test resulting from a loss of ligamentous support. Note the plantarflexion of rearfoot on the forefoot at the midtarsal joint.

eversion during terminal stance. This finding, as well as decreased hallux dorsiflexion in the AAF patients suggests a lack of loading of the first ray and failure to engage the windlass mechanism during heel rise.

The most significant finding of the study by Van de Velde and colleagues was the disruption of coupling or synchronized motion between the rearfoot and the forefoot, as well as the rearfoot and the lower leg in patients with PTTD, compared with healthy controls. Coupling is the mechanism where internal and external rotation of the leg is converted to inversion and eversion of the foot. Loss of coupling between skeletal segments has been theorized to be either the result or the cause of many musculoskeletal injuries.[79] A study of 11 injured runners showed out-of-phase coupling between the foot and leg, which was improved with use of custom orthotic devices.[80] Hintermann and associates,[81] in a cadaver study, showed a significant loss of coupling between the foot and leg when the medial ankle ligaments and the interosseous talocalcaneal ligament is severed, identical to what is seen in stage 3 AAF deformity. For the first time, an in vivo kinematic study from Van de Velde verified Hintermann's previous work, showing that the foot becomes mechanically disconnected from the leg when the medial ankle and arch ligaments are ruptured. The lack of connectivity or mechanical coupling between the foot and the leg poses one of several challenges in treating PTTD.

Orthotic Treatment of Posterior Tibial Tendon Dysfunction

There are 3 goals of treatment of PTTD: decrease pain, restore function and mobility, and prevent progression of the deformity. Orthotic treatment of PTTD can accomplish these 3 goals by restoring alignment and offloading the injured structures.

From gait and imaging studies, the AAF is characterized by 3 basic features: hindfoot valgus, collapse of the medial longitudinal arch, and forefoot abduction. Published kinematic studies reveal that orthotic devices can reduce this deformity via several mechanisms.

Imhauser and colleagues[82] used a static cadaver model of a flatfoot deformity to test how various orthotic devices could correct alignment. A custom molded University of California Berkeley Laboratory (UCBL) foot orthosis provided better correction of hindfoot eversion than the Arizona ankle-foot orthosis (AFO). The researchers proposed that the UCBL covered more surface area under the rearfoot and the plantarmedial arch area of the foot compared with the Arizona AFO and thus improved alignment better. This was not a dynamic gait study, however.

Another static cadaver flatfoot study was performed by Kitaoka and colleagues.[83] Two prefabricated foot orthoses (arch supports) were evaluated for improvement of alignment of a flatfoot model. Hindfoot valgus did not improve with either device and there was negligible improvement of arch height. Hirano and associates[84] studied a prefabricated foot orthosis to determine effects on gliding resistance of the TP tendon. This orthotic device again failed to restore alignment of a flatfoot model and also failed to reduce gliding resistance of the TP tendon created by the flatfoot model. Both studies show the futility of treating PTTD with prefabricated foot orthoses.

A follow-up study examining kinematics of healthy patients was carried out by Kitaoka and colleagues[85] evaluating rigid versus articulated (hinged) custom AFO braces. As expected, the rigid AFO devices limited sagittal ankle joint range of motion greater than the articulated device. However, the articulated AFO restricted motion across the midfoot joints to a greater degree than the rigid AFO devices. The articulated AFO also limited transverse plane motion across the midfoot better than the solid AFO. The authors suggested that, by limiting motion across the ankle joint, greater demand for motion was required at the midfoot joints. They also concluded that articulated AFOs would limit midfoot motion better than solid AFOs and this would be more desirable when using orthotic therapy to offload injured structures in the PTTD patient.

A comparison of 3 different types of ankle braces and effects on the kinematics of patients with PTTD was carried out in a series of studies by Neville and colleagues.[86–88] These studies measured foot motion and alignment in patients with stage 2 PTTD while wearing a custom solid gauntlet AFO, a custom articulated gauntlet AFO, a prefabricated air stirrup brace with inflatable bladder under the arch, and compared with the shoe only condition. The custom articulated AFO proved superior to the solid AFO in correcting hindfoot alignment in the frontal plane while the solid AFO provided better correction of medial longitudinal arch alignment. Both custom braces performed superior to the prefabricated ankle brace. None of the braces corrected forefoot abduction to any significant degree of correction.

To address the failure of AFOs to control forefoot abduction in patients with PTTD, Neville and colleagues[89] modified a solid AFO with an extension of the lateral support to just proximal to the fifth metatarsophalangeal joint. With an extended lateral flange, the solid AFO resisted all forefoot abduction and actually induced slight adduction motion of the forefoot.

Theoretically, an AFO has advantage over a foot orthosis by controlling tibial rotation. The AAF deformity is driven by a loss of integrity of the spring ligament complex as well as the deltoid ligament complex. Subluxation results in both the talonavicular and subtalar joints. The tibia and talus undergo significant internal rotation relative to the navicular as well as medial displacement relative to the calcaneus. The goal of orthotic intervention is to provide an effective restraint for tibial rotation, which then offloads the soft tissue structures affected by the subluxation seen in these joints (**Figs. 3** and **4**).

Further enhancement of frontal plane control of eversion of the hindfoot can be accomplished with a modification of the positive cast first described by Carlson and Berglund in 1979.[90] Carlson and Berglund describe a method to remove plaster from the positive cast beginning at the medial calcaneal tubercle and extending to the sustentaculum area of the cast. As much as 8 mm of plaster can be removed in this skive modification. The end result is a varus wedge shape induced into the hindfoot portion of the footplate of the brace to provide inversion moment to the subtalar joint (**Fig. 5**). Greater contour to the sustentaculum can enhance support to the talonavicular joint. No matter what casting technique is performed, the footplate of the

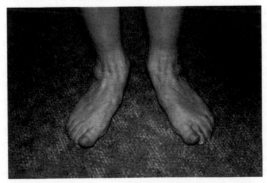

Fig. 3. Internal rotation of lower leg in right side stage 3 AAF, demonstrated by anterior displacement of the fibular malleolus. Note coupling of internal leg rotation with abduction of forefoot at talonavicular joint.

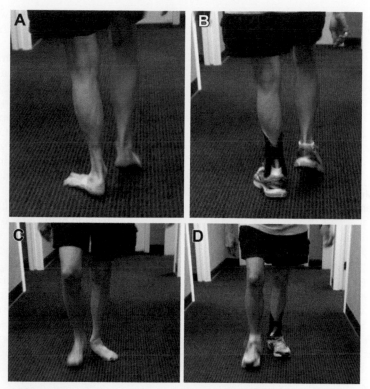

Fig. 4. An AFO can control tibial rotation in the transverse plane if it is adjusted with straps for tight fitting on the lower leg. (*A*) Back view without the AFO. (*B*) Back view with the AFO. (*C*) Front view without the AFO. (*D*) Front view with the AFO.

orthosis must tightly contour the plantar surface of the calcaneus to resist plantarflexion of the rearfoot, which is a common feature of the AAF.

Forefoot abduction can be controlled with the AFO via 2 mechanisms. Proximal control of internal tibial rotation is coupled with control of forefoot abduction across the midtarsal joint. Distally, the abducting forefoot can be restrained with an extended lateral flange (**Fig. 6**). Footwear becomes an important part of the brace system to control transverse plane motion of the foot.

The AAF is also characterized by dorsiflexion of the first metatarsal and inversion of the forefoot, induced by rearfoot eversion as well as sagittal plane collapse of the medial column. The footplate of the orthosis must conform to an everted or pronated forefoot, which is captured in the negative casting technique. The so-called forefoot supination deformity must be reduced in this casting procedure (**Fig. 7**).

CLINICAL STUDIES OF ORTHOTIC TREATMENT OF POSTERIOR TIBIAL TENDON DYSFUNCTION

Anecdotal reports of orthotic treatment of PTTD surfaced during the 1990s and consistently reported favorable outcomes, particularly when treating flexible stage 2 deformity.[91–95] The majority of these reports favored ankle bracing versus foot orthoses in terms of orthotic intervention for PTTD.

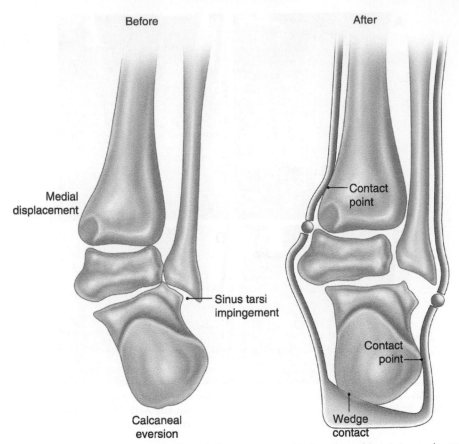

Fig. 5. Three key contact points will apply force above and below the ankle joint complex to correct alignment in the AAF deformity.

The lack of connectivity or mechanical coupling between the foot and the leg poses one of several challenges in treating PTTD. Foot orthoses primarily function by altering external moments acting on the joints of the lower extremity. This interaction depends on the coupling mechanisms operating between the foot and the leg. When these mechanisms are in place, foot orthoses can alter ground reaction forces at the plantar surface of the foot and affect transmission of torque to the proximal joints. When ligaments are disrupted in the AAF, these movement-coupling mechanisms are compromised and control of ankle and tibial rotation with foot orthoses is compromised. This proximal control of the hindfoot, ankle, and tibia can be better achieved with an AFO.

Notwithstanding, Kulig and colleagues[96] achieved significant reduction of pain using foot orthoses as part of an innovative rehabilitation program for patients in both stage 1 and stage 2 PTTD. Chao and colleagues[97] used a custom UCBL type foot orthosis treating stage 2 AAF and achieved excellent or good results in 70% of the patients. Custom foot orthoses seem to be effective and the intervention of choice when ligaments are intact, as seen in stage 1 and early stage 2 AAF deformity. Prefabricated foot orthoses show no effect on improving alignment of AAF.[83,84]

In clinical studies of stage 2 AAF, a variety of AFOs have achieved notable success in allowing patients to return to activity and avoid surgery.

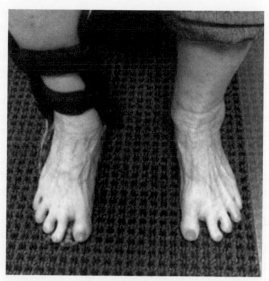

Fig. 6. Lateral flange must extend to fifth metatarsophalangeal joint to prevent abduction of forefoot.

Augustin and colleagues[98] prospectively studied 21 patients with stage 2 PTTD treated with a short custom-molded AFO (an Arizona brace). Despite a short follow-up period (mean, 12 months), they found significant changes in American Orthopaedic Foot and Ankle Society, Foot Function Index, and Short Form-36 scores. The American Orthopaedic Foot and Ankle Society score increased from 37.7 to 70.7. The Foot Function Index activity, pain, and disability scores improved to 14.8, 29.3, and 32.3, respectively.

Alvarez and coworkers[99] studied 47 consecutive patients with stage 1 or 2 PTTD in a nonoperative protocol combining orthoses with a structured rehabilitation program. A short articulated AFO was used if symptoms were present for more than 3 months and a three-quarter-length foot orthosis used if they were present less than 3 months. The median treatment period was 129 days with a minimum follow-up of 1 year. The average visual analogue scale was 1.0 after treatment. Among the patients, 89% were subjectively satisfied with their treatment, whereas 11% were dissatisfied and

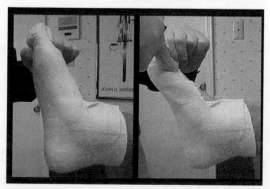

Fig. 7. Reducing forefoot supination deformity during casting process for orthosis.

went on to surgery. Only 8.5% of patients were unable to wean from the short articulated AFO. Therefore, 80.5% were successful in avoiding surgery and staying brace free.

Lin and colleagues[100] used a double metal upright AFO to treat stage 2 AAF in 32 patients. This study had an impressive follow-up of 8.6 years and 79% of the patients were brace free at that time and had avoided surgery. Overall, 94% of the patients were satisfied or partially satisfied. The researchers concluded that bracing has a high likelihood of avoiding surgery in AAF patients.

Krause and associates[101] used a shell brace, which was a modified supramalleolar AFO treating 18 patients with stage 2 PTTD. The clinical results were not as impressive as previous studies with true AFO braces. Irritation from the brace was seen in 16% of the patients and progression to stage 3 deformity was seen in another 16%. The remainder of the patients were satisfied at the 5-year follow-up with the results of the treatment with American Orthopaedic Foot and Ankle Society scores improving from baseline of 56 points to mean of 82 points.

Nielsen and coworkers[102] used a short articulated custom AFO to treat 64 patients with stage 2 AAF. With this brace, combined with physical therapy, 87.5% of the patients were able to avoid surgery over a 27-month observational period. The authors concluded: "Our interpretation of these findings is that bracing is, in general, a critical element of satisfactorily alleviating the symptoms of AAFD related to PTTD, and that use of the low articulating AFO may be particularly helpful because it combines a foot orthosis with support of the ankle, while enabling full weight-bearing ambulation."[102]

SUMMARY

The AAF deformity arises from attenuation and functional rupture of the posterior tibial tendon as well as the combined rupture of the spring ligament complex and the deltoid ligament complex. This deformity is characterized by hindfoot eversion, collapse of the medial longitudinal arch, and forefoot abduction. The pivotal joint in AAF is the talonavicular joint, destabilized by rupture of the spring ligament complex. The deformity at this joint is primarily accentuated in both the sagittal and the transverse plane. Frontal plane deformity occurs at both the ankle and the subtalar joints.

Orthotic management of AAF focuses on all 3 levels of the deformity. With loss of synchronous coupling between the foot and the leg, AFOs are preferred to control tibial rotation and thus control the talonavicular joint. Studies of treatment of AAF with various designs of AFO devices have demonstrated positive outcomes with more than 70% of patients avoiding surgery and functioning relatively pain free while also discontinuing use of their orthotic devices.

REFERENCES

1. Ross MH, Smith MD, Vicenzino B. Reported selection criteria for adult acquired flatfoot deformity and posterior tibial tendon dysfunction: are they one and the same? A systematic review. PLoS One 2017;12(12):e0187201.
2. Jahss MH. Spontaneous rupture of the tibialis posterior tendon: clinical findings. Tenographic studies and a new technique of repair. Foot Ankle 1982;3:158–66.
3. Johnson KA, Strom DE. Tibialis posterior tendon dysfunction. Clin Orthop 1989; 239:196–206.
4. Teasdall RD, Johnson KA. Surgical treatment of stage I posterior tibial tendon dysfunction. Foot Ankle Int 1994;15(12):646–8.
5. Downey DJ, Simpkin PA, Mack LA, et al. Tibialis posterior tendon rupture: a cause of rheumatoid flat foot. Arthritis Rheum 1988;31:441–4.

6. Michelson J, Easley M, Wigley FM, et al. Posterior tibial tendon dysfunction in rheumatoid arthritis. Foot Ankle Int 1995;16:156–61.

7. Myerson M, Solomon G, Shereff M. Posterior tibial tendon dysfunction: its association with seronegative disease. Foot Ankle 1989;9:219–25.

8. Richie DH. Biomechanics and clinical analysis of the adult acquired flatfoot. Clin Podiatr Med Surg 2007;24:617–44.

9. Myerson MS. Adult acquired flatfoot deformity: treatment of dysfunction of the posterior tibial tendon. Instr Course Lect 1997;46:393–405.

10. Funk DA, Cass JR, Johnson KA. Acquired adult flat foot secondary to posterior tibial-tendon pathology. J Bone Joint Surg Am 1986;68(1):95–102.

11. Dyal CM, Feder J, Deland JT, et al. Pes planus in patients with posterior tibial tendon insufficiency: asymptomatic versus symptomatic foot. Foot Ankle Int 1997;18:85–8.

12. Mann RA. Rupture of the tibialis posterior tendon. In: Instructional course lectures, American Academy of Orthopaedic Surgeons, vol. 33. St. Louis (MO): Mosby; 1982. p. 302–9.

13. Mueller TJ. Ruptures and lacerations of the tibialis posterior tendon. J Am Podiatry Assoc 1984;74(3):109–19.

14. Holmes GB II, Mann RA. Possible epidemiological factors associated with rupture of the posterior tibial tendon. Foot Ankle 1992;13:70–9.

15. Pomeroy GC, Pike RH, Beals TC, et al. Current concepts review. Acquired flatfoot in adults due to dysfunction of the posterior tibial tendon. J Bone Joint Surg 1999;81A:1173–82.

16. Lee MS, Vanore JV, Thomas JL, et al. Diagnosis and treatment of adult flatfoot. J Foot Ankle Surg 2005;44(2):78–113.

17. Morimoto I. Notes on architecture of tibialis posterior muscle in man. Kaibogaku Zasshi 1983;58:74–80.

18. Silver RL, de la Garza J, Rang M. The myth of muscle balance. J Bone Joint Surg 1985;67-B:432–7.

19. Kelikian AS, Sarrafian SK. Sarrafian's anatomy of the foot and ankle: descriptive, topographic, functional. Third edition. Philadelphia: Wolters Kluwer Health/Lippincott Williams & Wilkins; 2011.

20. Petersen W, Hohmann G, Pufe T, et al. Structure of the human tibialis posterior tendon. Arch Orthop Trauma Surg 2004;124(4):237–42.

21. Benjamin M, Ralphs JR. Fibrocartilage in tendons and ligaments and adaptation to compressive load. J Anat 1998;193:481–94.

22. Petersen W, Hohmann G, Stein V, et al. The blood supply of the posterior tibial tendon. J Bone Joint Surg Br 2002;84:141–4.

23. Stepien M. The sheath and arterial supply of the tendon of the posterior tibial muscle in man. Folia Morphol (Warsz) 1973;32:51–62.

24. Frey C, Shereff M, Greenidge N. Vascularity of the posterior tibial tendon. J Bone Joint Surg 1990;72-A:884–8.

25. Prado MP, Carvalho AE, Rodrigues CJ, et al. Vascular density of the posterior tibial tendon: a cadaver study. Foot Ankle Int 2006;27(8):628–31.

26. Deland JT, de Asla RJ, Sung IH, et al. Posterior tibial tendon insufficiency: which ligaments are involved? Foot Ankle Int 2005;26(6):427–35.

27. Deland JT, Arnoczky SP, Thompson FM. Adult acquired flatfoot deformity at the talonavicular joint: reconstruction of the spring ligament in an in vitro model. Foot Ankle Int 1992;13:327–32.

28. Davis WH, Sobel M, DiCarlo EF, et al. Gross, histological, and microvascular anatomy and biomechanical testing of the spring ligament complex. Foot Ankle Int 1996;17(2):95–102.
29. Patil V, Ebraheim NA, Frogameni A, et al. Morphometric dimensions of the calcaneonavicular (spring) ligament. Foot Ankle Int 2007;28(8):927–32.
30. Taniguchi A, Tanaka Y, Takakura Y, et al. Anatomy of the spring ligament. J Bone Joint Surg Am 2003;85-A(11):2174–8.
31. Vadell AM, Peratta M. Calcaneonavicular ligament: anatomy, diagnosis, and treatment. Foot Ankle Clin 2012;17:437–48.
32. Milner CE, Soames RW. The medial collateral ligaments of the human ankle joint: anatomical variations. Foot Ankle Int 1998;19(5):289–92.
33. Savage-Elliott I, Murawski CD, Smyth NA, et al. The deltoid ligament: an in-depth review of anatomy, function, and treatment strategies. Knee Surg Sports Traumatol Arthrosc 2013;21(6):1316–27.
34. Campbell KJ, Michalski MP, Wilson KJ, et al. The ligament anatomy of the deltoid complex of the ankle: a qualitative and quantitative anatomical study. J Bone Joint Surg Am 2014;96:e62.
35. Cromeens BP, Kirchhoff CA, Patterson RM, et al. An attachment-based description of the medial collateral and spring ligament complexes. Foot Ankle Int 2015; 36:710–21.
36. Amaha K, Nimura A, Yamaguchi R, et al. Anatomic study of the medial side of the ankle base on the joint capsule: an alternative description of the deltoid and spring ligament. J Exp Orthop 2019;6:2.
37. Kelly M, Masqoodi N, Vasconcellos D, et al. Spring ligament tear decreases static stability of the ankle joint. Clin Biomech 2019;61:79–83.
38. Sutherland DN. An electromyographic study of the plantar flexors of the ankle in normal walking on the level. J Bone Joint Surg Am 1966;48A:66–7.
39. Hintermann B, Nigg BM, Sommer C. Foot movement and tendon excursion: an in vitro study. Foot Ankle Int 1994;15:386–95.
40. McCullough MB, Ringleb SI, Arai K, et al. Moment arms of the ankle throughout the range of motion in three planes. Foot Ankle Int 2011;32(3):301–7.
41. Wickiewicz TL, Roy RR, Powell PL, et al. Muscle Architecture of the human lower limb. Clin Orthop Rel Res 1983;179:317–25.
42. Hui HJ, Beals TC, Brown NT. Influence of tendon transfer site on moment arms of the flexor digitorum longus muscle. Foot Ankle Int 2007;28(4).
43. Kohls-Gatzoulis J, Angel JC, Singh D, et al. Tibialis posterior dysfunction: a common and treatable cause of adult acquired flatfoot. BMJ 2004;329(7478): 1328–33.
44. Williams G, Widnall J, Evans P, et al. Could failure of the spring ligament complex be the driving force behind the development of the adult flatfoot deformity? J Foot Ankle Surg 2014;53(2):152–5.
45. Pasapula C, Cutts S. Modern theory of the development of adult acquired flat foot and an updated spring ligament classification system. Clin Res Foot Ankle 2017;5(3):247.
46. Tao K, Ji W-T, Wang D-M, et al. Relative contributions of plantar fascia and ligaments on the arch static stability: a finite element study. Biomed Tech Biomed Eng 2010;55:265–71.
47. Huang CK, Kitaoka HB, An KN, et al. Biomechanical evaluation of longitudinal arch stability. Foot Ankle 1993;14(6):353–7.
48. Kitaoka HB, Luo ZP, An KN. Three-dimensional analysis of flatfoot deformity: cadaver study. Foot Ankle Int 1998;19(7):447–51.

49. Chu IT, Myerson MS, Nyska M, et al. Experimental flatfoot model: the contribution of dynamic loading. Foot Ankle Int 2001;22(3):220–5.

50. Jennings MM, Christensen JC. The effects of sectioning the spring ligament on rear foot stability and posterior tibial tendon efficiency. Foot Ankle Surg 2008; 47(3):219–24.

51. De la Portilla CC, Larrainzar-Garijo R, Bayod J. Biomechanical stress analysis of the main soft tissues associated with the development of adult acquired flatfoot deformity. Clin Biomech 2019;61(1):163–71.

52. Jahss MH. Tendon disorders of the foot and ankle. In: Jahss MH, editor. Disorders of the foot and ankle. Medical and surgical management. Philadelphia: W. B. Saunders; 1991. p. 1461–513.

53. Murley GS, Menz HB, Landorf KB. Foot posture influences the electromyographic activity of selected lower limb muscles during gait. J Foot Ankle Res 2009;2:35.

54. Gray EG, Basmajian JV. Electromyography and cinematography of leg and foot ("normal" and flat) during walking. Anat Rec 1968;161:1–15.

55. Keenan MA, Peabody JK, Perry J. Valgus deformities of the feet and characteristics of gait in patients who have rheumatoid arthritis. J Bone Joint Surg Am 1991;73:237–47.

56. An KN, Berglund L, Uchiyama S, et al. Measurement of friction between pulley and flexor tendon. Biomed Sci Instrum 1993;29:1–7.

57. Zhao C, Amadio PC, Zobitz ME, et al. Gliding resistance after repair of partially lacerated human flexor digitorum profundus tendon in vitro. Clin Biomech (Bristol, Avon) 2001;16:696–701.

58. Uchiyama E, Kitaoka HB, Fujii T, et al. Gliding resistance of the posterior tibial tendon. Foot Ankle Int 2006;27(9):723–6.

59. Arai K, Ringleb SI, Zhao KD, et al. The effect of flatfoot deformity and tendon loading on the work of friction measured in the posterior tibial tendon. Clin Biomech 2007;22:592–8.

60. Fujii T, Uchiyama E, Kitaoka HB, et al. The influence of flatfoot deformity on the gliding resistance of tendons about the ankle. Foot Ankle Int 2009;30(11): 1107–10.

61. McCormack AP, Ching RP, Sangeorzan BJ. Biomechanics of procedures used in adult flatfoot deformity. Foot Ankle Clin 2001;6:15–23.

62. Reeck J, Felten N, McCormack AP, et al. Support of the talus: a biomechanical investigation of the contributions of the talonavicular and talocalcaneal joints, and the superomedial calcaneonavicular ligament. Foot Ankle Int 1998;19: 674–82.

63. Balen PF, Helms CA. Association of posterior tibial tendon injury with spring ligament injury, sinus tarsi abnormality, and plantar fasciitis on MR imaging. Am J Roentgenol 2001;176:1137–43.

64. Ormsby N, Jackson G, Evans P, et al. Imaging of the tibionavicular ligament and its potential role in Adult Acquired Flatfoot deformity. Foot Ankle Int 2018;39(5): 629–35.

65. Johnson JE, Harris GF. Pathomechanics of posterior tibial tendon insufficiency. Foot Ankle Clin 1997;2:227–39.

66. Myerson MS. Adult acquired flatfoot deformity. Treatment of dysfunction of the posterior tibial tendon. J Bone Joint Surg 1996;78-A:780–92.

67. Phillips RD, Phillips RL. Quantitative analysis of the locking position of the midtarsal joint. J Am Podiatry Assoc 1983;73(10):518–22.

68. Gatt A, Chockalingam N, Chevalier TL. Sagittal plane kinematics of the foot during passive ankle dorsiflexion. Prosthet Orthot Int 2011;35:425–31.

69. Blackwood CB, Yuen TJ, Sangeorzan BJ, et al. The midtarsal joint locking mechanism. Foot Ankle Int 2005;26:1074–80.

70. Gazdag AR, Cracchiolo A III. Rupture of the posterior tibial tendon. Evaluation of injury of the spring ligament and clinical assessment of tendon transfer and ligament repair. J Bone Joint Surg 1997;79-A:675–81.

71. Rattanaprasert U, Smith R, Sullivan M, et al. Three-dimensional kinematics of the forefoot, rearfoot, and leg without the function of tibialis posterior in comparison with normals during stance phase of walking. Clin Biomech 1999;14:14–23.

72. Tome J, Nawoczenski DA, Flemister A, et al. Comparison of foot kinematics between subjects with posterior tibialis tendon dysfunction and healthy controls. J Orthop Sports Phys Ther 2006;36:635–44.

73. Ringleb SI, Kavros SJ, Kotajarvi BR, et al. Changes in gait associated with acute stage II posterior tibial tendon dysfunction. Gait Posture 2007;25:555–64.

74. Houck JR, Neville CG, Tome J, et al. Ankle and foot kinematics associated with stage II PTTD during stance. Foot Ankle Int 2009;30(6):530–9.

75. Ness ME, Long J, Marks R, et al. Foot and ankle kinematics in patients with posterior tibial tendon dysfunction. Gait Posture 2008;27:331–9.

76. Neville C, Flemister AS, Houck J. Total and distributed plantar loading in subjects with stage II tibialis posterior tendon dysfunction during terminal stance. Foot Ankle Int 2013;34:131–9.

77. Neville C, Flemister AS, Houck JR. Deep posterior compartment strength and foot kinematics with stage II posterior tibial tendon dysfunction. Foot Ankle Int 2010;31(4):320–8.

78. Van de Velde M, Matricali GA, Wuite S, et al. Foot segmental motion and coupling in stage II and III tibialis posterior tendon dysfunction. Clin Biomech 2017;45:38–42.

79. Chuter VH, Janse de Jonge XAK. Proximal and distal contributions to lower extremity injury: a review of the literature. Gait Posture 2012;36:7–15.

80. Ferber R, McClay Davis I, Williams DS III. Effect of foot orthotics on rearfoot and tibia joint coupling patterns and variability. J Biomech 2005;38:477–83.

81. Hintermann B, Sommer C, Nigg B. Influence of ligament transection on tibial and calcaneal rotation with loading and dorsiflexion – plantarflexion. Foot and Ankle 1995;16:567–71.

82. Imhauser CW, Abidi NA, Frankel DZ, et al. Biomechanical evaluation of the efficacy of external stabilizers in the conservative treatment of acquired flatfoot deformity. Foot Ankle Int 2002;23:727–37.

83. Kitaoka HB, Luo ZP, Kura H, et al. Effect of foot orthoses on 3-dimensional kinematics of flatfoot: a cadaveric study. Arch Phys Med Rehabil 2002;83:876–9.

84. Hirano T, McCullough MBA, Kitaoka HB, et al. Effects of foot orthoses on the work of friction of the posterior tibial tendon. Clin Biomech 2009;24:776–80.

85. Kitaoka HB, Crevoisier XM, Harbst K, et al. The effect of custom-made braces for the ankle and hindfoot on ankle and foot kinematics and ground reaction forces. Arch Phys Med Rehabil 2006;87:130–5.

86. Neville C, Flemister AS, Houck JR. Effects of the AirLift PTTD brace on foot kinematics in subjects with stage II posterior tibial tendon dysfunction. J Orthop Sports Phys Ther 2009;39:201–9.

87. Neville C, Houck J. Choosing among 3 ankle-foot orthoses for a patient with stage II posterior tibial tendon dysfunction. J Orthop Sports Phys Ther 2009; 39:816–24.

88. Neville C, Lemley FR. Effect of ankle-foot orthotic devices on foot kinematics in Stage II posterior tibial tendon dysfunction. Foot Ankle Int 2012;33:406–14.
89. Neville C, Bucklin M, Ordway N, et al. An ankle-foot orthosis with a lateral extension reduces forefoot abduction in subjects with stage II posterior tibial tendon dysfunction. Orthop Sports Phys Ther 2016;46(1):26–33.
90. Carlson JM, Berglund G. An effective orthotic design for controlling the unstable subtalar joint. Orthotics and Prosthetics 1979;33(1):39–49.
91. Logue JD. Advances in orthotics and bracing. Foot Ankle Clin 2007;12:215–32.
92. Bek N, Öznur A, Kavlak Y, et al. The effect of orthotic treatment of posterior tibial tendon insufficiency on pain and disability. Pain Clin 2003;15:345–50.
93. Marzano R, Marzano R. Functional bracing of the adult acquired flatfoot. Clin Podiatr Med Surg 2007;24:645–56.
94. Noll KH. The use of orthotic devices in adult acquired flatfoot deformity. Foot Ankle Clin 2001;6:25–36.
95. Steb HS, Marzano R. Conservative management of posterior tibial tendon dysfunction, subtalar joint complex, and pes planus deformity. Clin Podiatr Med Surg 1999;16:439–51.
96. Kulig K, Reischl SF, Pomrantz AB, et al. Smith RW Nonsurgical management of posterior tibial tendon dysfunction with orthoses and resistive exercise: a randomized controlled trial. Phys Ther 2009;89:26–37.
97. Chao W, Wapner KL, Lee TH, et al. Non-operative management of posterior tibial tendon dysfunction. Foot Ankle Int 1996;17(12):736–41.
98. Augustin JF, Lin SS, Berberian WS, et al. Non-operative treatment of adult acquired flat foot with the Arizona brace. Foot Ankle Clin 2003;8(3):491–502.
99. Alvarez RG, Marini A, Schmitt C, et al. Stage I and II posterior tibial tendon dysfunction treated by a structured non-operative management protocol: an orthosis and exercise program. Foot Ankle Int 2006;27(1):2–8.
100. Lin JL, Balbas J, Richardson EG. Results of non-surgical treatment of stage II posterior tibial tendon dysfunction: a 7- to 10-year followup. Foot Ankle Int 2008;29(8):525–30.
101. Krause F, Bosshard A, Lehmann O, et al. Shell brace for stage II posterior tibial tendon insufficiency. Foot Ankle Int 2008;29(11):1095–100.
102. Nielsen MD, Dodson EE, Shadrick DL, et al. Non-operative care for the treatment of adult-acquired flatfoot deformity. J Foot Ankle Surg 2011;50:311–4.

Biomechanical Effects of Shoe Gear on the Lower Extremity

Scott Spencer, DPM

KEYWORDS

- Shoe gear • Lower extremity • Foot

KEY POINTS

- The information gleaned from kinetic and kinematic studies on foot function and gait in relation to shoes can be applied clinically after considering the key findings of the research discussed in this article.
- These studies demonstrate the events of the gait cycle are somewhat different from what many providers have been taught.
- Greater pronation of the subtalar joint when entering the propulsive period, where resupination will most likely be occurring, would be expected.

INTRODUCTION

Shoes are an ever-evolving entity. As a society, they are worn to convey status, athletic ability, fashion sense, activity and for foot health. With the broad range of different shoe types and styles, it has become increasingly difficult to know which shoes are beneficial, whether for everyday wear or for activity-specific wear.

Although every practitioner has shoes that they are comfortable recommending to patients, many may not be fully aware of the consequences to gait brought on by the shoes. It is easy to tell a patient not to wear a certain type of shoe based on common sense. It is important for the care provider to have an understanding, however, as to why a shoe or a feature of a shoe is not conducive to a healthy gait or may be contributing to the development of pathology.

A good adjunct to this article was written by Fuller in 1994.[1] In this article, Fuller discussed the components of shoes that should be taken into account when assessing or recommending a shoe to a patient. A similarly helpful contribution comes from Snijders in 1987,[2] where he described different elements of the stance phase of the gait cycle and explained the effects of shoes during these time periods.

Disclosures: None.
Department of Surgery/Biomechanics, Kent State University College of Podiatric Medicine, 6000 Rockside Woods Boulevard, Independence, OH 44131, USA
E-mail address: Sspenc16@kent.edu

In 2013, Farber and Knudson[3] surveyed 866 orthopedists and reported on 276 responses regarding shoe recommendations; 64% recommended New Balance athletic shoes whereas 26% did not recommend specific brands; 50% of the respondents wore New Balance, whereas 25% wore Nike. With respect to dress shoes, 27% recommended Rockport and 27% recommended SAS; 76% of respondents were familiar with the American Orthopaedic Foot & Ankle Society shoe fit guidelines, with only 56% educating their patients on these guidelines and 43% giving no consideration to the idea that patients may take into account the practitioners' shoes when selecting their own shoe. This variability in prescribing patterns highlights the importance of understanding the biomechanical effects of shoes on gait.

With the advent of many specialized shoes claiming to strengthen muscles and create greater efficiency of gait, the practitioner must sort through many options. The purpose of this article is to provide the foot health care provider with a better understanding of the effects of shoes on the mechanics of gait based on recent literature.

FOOT MECHANICS

The first point of understanding for any discussion of shoes and their effects on gait should be the mechanics of the foot. With the advent of better foot segment modeling, researchers are able to observe and quantify the motions of the foot utilizing markers and multicamera gait analysis systems. Researchers are also better able to measure forces and center of progression of the foot during gait, both barefoot and shod. Kitaoka and Crevoisier,[4] using segment modeling, were able to analyze calcaneal-tibial and metatarsal-calcaneal movement in all 3 body planes while also utilizing a force plate to obtain ground reactive force data.

Their results showed that for the 20 healthy subjects tested the cadence averaged 109.15 steps ± 7.05 steps per minute, with the gait cycle lasting an average of 1.11 seconds ± 0.07 seconds, the average stance phase taking 0.70 seconds ± 0.06 seconds, and a stance phase percentage of 63.07% ± 1.74%. With respect to motion in the sagittal plane, heel strike was perpendicular to slightly dorsiflexed, followed by rapid plantarflexion. Although the investigators did not break the events observed into periods of the stance phase of gait, it seems that in the midstance period of gait the foot dorsiflexed 6.5° ± 2.7°. The propulsive period saw plantarflexion of the foot of 11.8° ± degrees.[4]

Notably, in the frontal plane, the rearfoot everted relative to the leg at heel contact and late into the stance phase and inverted until the end of the stance phase.[4] This differed from the idea of rearfoot inversion occurring earlier in the stance phase of gait and suggested the subtalar joint did not actually supinate until heel off during the propulsive period of the gait cycle. This author has made similar observations over the years.

When the investigators examined the metatarsal to calcaneus relationship in the sagittal plane, they found the midfoot slightly plantarflexed at heel strike with gradual dorsiflexion late in stance followed by plantarflexion until the end of the stance phase. In the frontal plane, the forefoot was in a rectus position at heel strike, then everting until late in the stance phase. This corresponded with the rearfoot motion observed. In the transverse plane the forefoot was internally rotated at heel strike, externally rotated, and then internally rotated again until the end of the stance phase of the gait cycle.[4]

Vertical ground reactive force increased during the contact period, decreased during the midstance period and then increased again during the propulsive period.[4] A difference from the commonly taught vertical ground reactive force graph was that the first peak was slightly higher than the second peak in vertical ground reactive force. An observation was that the medial-lateral ground reactive forces were maintained medially for the vast majority of the stance phase of gait.

HEEL HEIGHT AND ITS EFFECT ON GAIT

Height differential is present in the vast majority of shoes worn today. From running shoes to dress shoes and almost everything in between, heel height has a significant effect on patients. What, then, does the literature reveal about the impact of heel height on patients' feet and the resulting mechanical changes that can be anticipated (summarized in **Box 1**)?

In 2013, Yu and colleagues[5] simulated walking with high-heeled shoes and noted several findings related to women's high-heeled shoes. In this study, the simulations looked at a women's shoes with a 2-in heel height and a narrow toe area with a squared distal aspect, mirroring what some perceive to be a sensible women's dress shoe. The authors incorporated into their simulation the findings from an American Orthopedic & and Ankle Society 1993 study, which found 88% of women wear shoes that were smaller than their feet.[6]

The investigators found that simply donning the simulated shoe resulted in lateral deviation of the hallux and varus rotation of the fifth digit. The study also found that there were small areas of peak pressure during heel strike and propulsion, with plantar pressure greatest under the first, second, and third metatarsal heads. With respect to dorsal pressure, there was increased contact pressure on the dorsal medial aspect of the hallux, with little increase noted across the rest of the digits. When simulating propulsion, the investigators found a much higher hallux valgus angle relative to the varus angle of the fifth digit. With respect to the stress on the metatarsals during propulsion, the greatest stress was on the second and third metatarsals.

A literature review by Cronin[7] and an article by Wiedemeijer and Otten[8] highlighted some of the effects of high-heeled shoes on gait. The investigators pointed out that between 37% and 69% of women wear what could be classified as high-heeled shoes on a daily basis. High-heeled shoes were defined as any shoe where the heel was higher than the forefoot area, possibly having a heel elevation of up to 10 cm, and often including a narrow toe box, rigid heel cap, and a curved plantar region.

Biomechanically, the effects of high-heeled shoes on gait were a slower walking speed with shorter strides, without a change in cadence.[9] There was increased energy expenditure measured when walking on a treadmill. The center of mass was moved

---

Box 1
High-heeled shoe effects on gait

1. Compression of toes
2. Medial vertical ground reactive force increase
3. Increase hallux halgus angle relative to varus angle of fifth digit
4. Decrease in walking speed
5. Increased energy expenditure
6. Increased frictional demands on the forefoot
7. Long-term wear resulting in arch flattening
8. Acquired equinus

anteriorly and superiorly, which led to knee flexion and increased lower limb muscle activity. A finding was an increased plantar friction demand, which suggested an increased likelihood of slipping on lower friction surfaces. The impact on ground reactive forces in high-heeled shoe wear was to create a greater deceleration demand for the center of mass and, therefore, an increased demand for acceleration of the center of mass for propulsion, resulting in a decrease in the fluidity of gait. This created greater shock at impact, which may cause soft tissue damage in the spine and lower extremity. A finding was that when heel height was increased from 7.6 cm to 8.5 cm, the impact force and load rate both decreased.

The effects of high-heeled shoes on the spine were mixed. There was debate regarding increased lordosis, with the general conclusion that there was no increase.[10,11] There was an increase, however, in erector spinae muscle activity, with the investigators suggesting this activity may result in increased spinal compression over time. There may have been an increase in hip flexor movement early in the gait cycle, but no appreciable effect on the hip was noted.[12] With respect to the knee, there was increased knee flexion, which caused quadricep activation and increased patellofemoral stress anteriorly.

The observations of increased loading rate for the first metatarsal and decreased loading rate for the fifth metatarsal were observed, as discussed previously, leading to a possible correlation between heel height and hallux valgus.

In 2014 Lee and Li[13] examined asymmetric load carrying with high heels during walking. These researchers sought to identify if activities, such as carrying a purse, would have an impact on gait in high-heeled shoes. They found that all of the previously mentioned findings were increased with the addition of the asymmetric load.

The long-term implications of wearing high-heeled shoes were explored in 2 articles. Pan and colleagues[14] in 2016 used a control group who had not worn heels and then grouped subjects into wear durations of less than 2 years, 2 years to 5 years, 6 years to 10 years, 11 years to 20 years, and longer than 20 years. The study showed that in the 2-year to 5-year group, the longitudinal arch elevated, but in the 6-year to 10-year group the longitudinal arch flattened, whereas in the 20 years and above group, the forefoot transverse arch tended to collapse.

Anecdotally, it is commonplace for providers to place a patient who was a long-term high-heeled shoe wearer in what was perceived to be a sensible shoe, only to have the patient reject the shoe due to discomfort. Kim and colleagues[15] found that the dorsiflexion range of motion in subjects who were long-standing high-heeled shoe wearers was decreased relative to non–high-heeled shoe wearers, indicating acquired equinus. Perhaps more interesting was that inversion strength of the foot was decreased and eversion strength was increased in these long-term high-heel–wearing subjects, indicating a possible decrease over time in the posterior tibialis strength and increase in the strength of the fibularis brevis (see **Box 1**).

GENERAL EFFECT OF SHOES ON FOOT FUNCTION

With the advent of many different types of shoes, such as zero drop, 4-mm drop, minimalist, and standard durometer hard-soled shoes, it is difficult to know the effect of different variations of shoe construction on foot function. Thus, a discussion about the research that addressed various components of the shoe and how these components influence foot function is beneficial (summarized in **Table 1**).

Rao and colleagues[16] examined 8 male runners who had worn standard running shoes but had not run in minimalist running shoes. Three-dimensional kinematics were assessed utilizing motion analysis that produced anywhere from 1° to 3° of

Table 1	
Summarized effects of shoes on foot function	
Shoe Characteristic	**Effect on Function**
Changing from classic to minimalist shoe gear	• Forefoot-first strike pattern • Greater diffusion of plantar forces • Reduced hip and knee rotation moments
Improper fitting pediatric shoe gear	• Digital deformities and improper forefoot loading
Unshod benefits in children	• Increased proprioception, strength, and decreased planus deformity
Shoe effects in frontal and transverse planes	• Increased ability to constrain the foot in these planes
Importance of proper flex point	• MTPJ location is variable and more important in rigid-soled shoes
Effect on stride length	• Increased stride length when shod and decreased when barefoot
Ankle plantarflexion	• Decreased when wearing shoes and increased when barefoot
Windlass mechanism	• Increased in high-heeled shoes causing greater forefoot plantar pressures • Decreased in all other shoe types
COP	• Reduced peak ground reactive forces • Reduced COP excursion

freedom with respect to motion at various joints, including the ankle, knee, and hip joints. Electromyographic (EMG) data of the anterior tibialis, posterior tibialis, gastrocnemius, and fibularis muscles also were obtained. The subjects were then analyzed running barefoot, in a minimalist shoe, and in a classic-thickness shoe at a speed of 12 km per hour. The investigators found no significant difference with changing footwear when looking at the EMG, joint kinematics, or the torque at the joints when comparing classic running shoes to minimalist running shoes. The study corroborated earlier research when comparing shod to barefoot running, demonstrating a natural midfoot or forefoot-first striking pattern. The study found no difference between the physiologic or mechanical responses during the stance phase of running with the shod runners. The investigators did relate that this was probably due to adaptation of running style and that long-term studies of the adaptation needed to be carried out.

This is important in runners who switch from traditional shoes to more minimalist shoes and barefoot running, where there is a change in the foot strike pattern, with barefoot and minimalist shoes showing a forefoot-first strike pattern or midfoot pattern. This is a change that any patient considering minimalist or barefoot running must employ to avoid injury.

Kurup and colleagues[17] provided a review of the various shoe permutations that might be encountered. They looked at shoe gear in children, with the observation that shoes that are too small increase the hallux valgus angle, causing lesser toe deformities, whereas adding increased heel height activated the windlass mechanism, leading to abnormal forefoot loading. They also noted the work of Rao and Joseph, who found a flatfoot in 8.6% of shod children as opposed to 2.8% in children who did not wear shoes. These observations highlight the importance of monitoring shoe size in growing children and may illustrate the potential benefit of barefoot walking via an increased proprioception incurred by the unshod foot. These observations were noted with respect to different variations of shoes, such as negative heel shoes, flip-flops, and All Phases of Step shoes. This highlights the possible benefit of children spending time barefoot to enhance proprioception and strengthen the foot.

Morio and colleagues[18] studied footwear's effect on movement of the forefoot relative to the rearfoot during both walking and running. The investigators used multisegment foot modeling and a specially created sandal to attempt to demonstrate the restrictive effect of shoes on the foot. The investigators analyzed the subjects walking barefoot, shod with a sandal consisting of a soft midsole, and shod with a sandal consisting of a hard midsole. The study demonstrated that motion was constrained in the frontal and transverse planes but not in the sagittal plane. This effect was greater in walking than in running. This implies the potential for exerting better control of feet in the frontal or transverse planes with the use of shoes.

In the past, consumers had their shoe size and width measured utilizing a Brannock device. This instrument not only measured the length of the foot with respect to the toes but also with respect to the flexion point of the first metatarsophalangeal joint (MTPJ). A study by Thompson[19] and colleagues looked the location of the first MTPJ and the location of forefoot bend, focusing on general-purpose women's footwear. The investigators found that the first MTPJ flexion point ranged from 70% to 79% of the total foot length in the test subjects, whereas the latest design specifications cited by the investigators showed a flexion point for the first MTPJ at between 63% and 66%, demonstrating a discrepancy. Based on these findings, an important measurement to obtain is the first MTPJ flexion point in shoes that have more rigid soles and suggest purchasing more flexible soled shoes to prevent abnormal shearing forces, strain reduction, and injury.

Perhaps the best way to view the effects of shoes on mechanical function of the foot is to look at comparisons between shod subjects and unshod subjects. Two relatively recent studies have examined the effects on gait biomechanics under these circumstances, with one adding a popular warm weather footwear style, the flip-flop.

Franklin and colleagues[20] in 2015 reviewed studies that assessed kinetics, kinematics, and muscle activity between barefoot walking and commonly worn footwear. In the course of their review, they found a reduction in barefoot gait velocity in studies where the participants wore their own shoes as opposed to the prescribed study shoes. Stride length was reduced with barefoot walking that increased with flexible shoes. An increase in ankle joint plantarflexion also was noted in the barefoot walkers. When looking at studies involving habitual barefoot walkers and shod walkers, it was noted that the barefoot participants had anatomically larger forefoot areas and an initial flatter foot placement when walking, which had the effect of reducing pressure on the foot by spreading out the distribution of the plantar force placed on the foot. This was opposed to shoe wearers, who were not able to spread forces as evenly across the foot.

Another product of a decreased stride length in barefoot walking is the effect on joints other than the foot during gait. Franklin and colleagues[20] observed a reduction in hip flexor and extensor and knee varus moments, with an increase in knee flexor moment. These areas are all associated with the formation of osteoarthritis. The investigators asserted that heel height in shoes contributed to the knee varus moments. The forefoot spreading while barefoot, and the restriction of this when shod, was evidenced in pediatric studies, with a correlation between shoe wear and the development of foot problems later in life. Franklin and colleagues[20] hypothesized that wearing shoes led to a decrease in function of the windlass mechanism due to restriction in lengthening of the foot during gait when shod. Another correlation was noted between the variety of shoes worn, placing the foot in unnatural positions during shod walking with an impact on arch height and ultimately weakening the foot contributing to pedal pathology.

Zhang and colleagues[21] in 2013 looked at gait effects in 4 different scenarios: wearing a running shoe, wearing a sandal comparable to what today might be referred to as a slide, wearing a more traditional flip-flop with the attachment point in the first interspace and straps across the dorsal aspect of the metatarsals, and barefoot. Regarding stance time, the study's findings were the same as discussed previously, with the shortest being barefoot and the longest being the running shoe. The first peak in vertical ground reactive forces and peak propulsive ground reactive forces were lower in shoes than barefoot or either sandal. These researchers additionally found greater medial to lateral displacement while barefoot, followed by sandals, and finally shoes. Anteroposterior displacement, however, was less when barefoot compared with the shod options. These findings are most likely related to the increasing restriction on the foot by shoe gear and the shorter strides taken while barefoot. The remaining ankle, knee, and hip effects were similar to those discussed previously.

These studies demonstrate the effect of shoes on foot function. Wearing shoes increases stride length, decreases ankle joint plantarflexion, and constrains the forefoot, altering the ability to distribute force across the metatarsal heads. Shoes also seem to have a negative impact on the windlass mechanism during gait, with joint motions of the hip and knee increased with shoe wear. Advantageously, shoes tend to reduce peaks in ground reactive forces, and reduce the excursion of the center of pressure (COP) during gait, which may or may not be a benefit for patients and their balance (see **Table 1**).

SHOE INSTABILITY EFFECT ON GAIT

For a time, manufactured instability in shoes was a popular trend. This instability acts as a model, providing insight into potential implications of shoes that have worn out. Every practitioner has seen a patient who has worn shoes well past the shoe's life expectancy, no doubt aggravating the patient's pathology.

Nigg and colleagues[22] in 2006 examined the Masai Barefoot Technology shoe. The study examined kinetics, kinematics, and muscle activity in both standing and walking environments. While standing, the COP excursion was greater in the unstable shoe than the more stable control. Muscle activity was increased most significantly for the tibialis anterior muscle. Kinematically, in the unstable shoe the ankle joint was more dorsiflexed in the first half of stance than the stable shoe, correlating with the noted increase in anterior tibialis function when standing. There were no significant kinetic differences between the stable and unstable shoes. With respect to EMG, there were no significant differences noted, but a reduction in EMG activity was found in the stable shoe control.

Khoury and colleagues[23] in 2013 studied the COP trajectory with alterations to the sole of a shoe. Using a shoe that allowed the researchers to alter medial and lateral pressure applied to the foot via the sole of the shoe, the investigators used in-shoe pressure data to measure these pressures during different periods of the stance phase of gait. The study demonstrated that the COP trajectory shifted with the differing medial or lateral loading introduced to the sole of the shoe. Increases in lateral pressure moved the COP medially and medial pressure moved the COP more lateral.

The significance of these studies may best be applied to shoes that are exhibiting wear patterns that deform and or destabilize the shoe, as in shoes that are worn past their useful lives. Materials in the soles of shoes deform over time and with excessive use. This may cause increased demand on musculature to establish stability while also shifting the COP away from what is healthy for the patient, resulting in altered force distribution during gait and causing stress to soft tissue and osseous structures, resulting in pathology.

SUMMARY

The information gleaned from kinetic and kinematic studies on foot function and gait in relation to shoes can be applied clinically after considering the key findings of the research discussed in this article. These studies demonstrate the events of the gait cycle are somewhat different from what many providers have been taught. Greater protonation of the subtalar joint when entering the propulsive period, where resupination will most likely be occurring, would be expected to be seen. The midfoot seems to follow what has been traditionally thought with respect to motion during gait. Ground reactive forces also follow the traditional curve, with peaks at the end of the contact period and shortly after entering the propulsive period.

The importance of having an understanding of the effects of shoes on the foot function during gait cannot be underestimated and should be incorporated into every pedal evaluation conducted on a patient. By making shoe assessment a habit and understanding the effects shoes can have on the foot during gait, providers can better tailor treatment plans to maximize outcomes, while giving patients greater insight into the possible negative effects their choice of shoes may have on foot function.

REFERENCES

1. Fuller E. A review of the biomechanics of shoes. Clin Podiatr Med Surg 1994; 11(2):241–58.
2. Snijders CJ. Biomechanics of footwear. Clin Podiatr Med Surg 1987;4(3):629–44.
3. Farber DC, Knulsen EJ. Footwear recommendations and patterns among orthopaedic foot and ankle surgeons. Foot and Ankle Spec 2013;8(6):457–64.
4. Kitaoka HB, Crevoisier XM. Foot and ankle kinematics and ground reaction forces during ambulation. Foot Ankle Int 2006;27(10):808–13.
5. Yu J, Cheung J, Wong D, et al. Biomechanical simulation of high-heeled shoe donning and walking. J Biomech 2013;46:2067–74.
6. Thompson F, Coughlin M. The high price of high-fashion footwear. Instr Course Lect 1995;44:371–7.
7. Cronin NJ. The effects of high heeled shoes on female gait: a review. J Electromyogr Kinesiol 2014;24:258–63.
8. Wiedemeijer MM, Otten E. Effects of high heeled shoes on gait. A review. Gait Posture 2018;61:423–30.
9. Sipio E, Piccini G, Pecchioli C, et al. Walking variations in healthy women wearing high-heeled shoes: shoe size and heel height effects. Gait Posture 2018;63: 195–201.
10. Schroeder J, Hallander K. Effects of high-heeled footwear on static and dynamic pelvis position and lumber lordosis in experiences younger and middle aged women. Gait Posture 2018;59:53–7.
11. Baaklini E, Angst M, Schellenberg F, et al. High-heeled walking decreases lumbar lordosis. Gait Posture 2017;55:12–4.
12. Mika A, Clark BC, Lesky L. The influence of high and low heeled shoes on EMG timing characteristics of the lumbar and hip extensor complex during trunk forward flexion and return task. Man Ther 2013;18(6):506–11.

13. Lee S, Li JX. Effects of high-heeled shoes and asymmetrical load carrying on lower extremity kinematics during walking in young women. J Am Podiatr Med Assoc 2014;104(1):58–65.
14. Yin CM, Pan XH, Sun YX, et al. Effects of duration of wearing high-heeled shoes on plantar pressure. Hum Mov Sci 2016;49:196–205.
15. Kim Y, Lim JM, Yoon BC. Changes in ankle range of motion and muscle strength in habitual wearers of high-heeled shoes. Foot Ankle Int 2013;34(3):414–9.
16. Rao G, Chambon N, Gueguen N, et al. Does wearing shoes affect your biomechanical efficiency? J Biomech 2015;48:413–7.
17. Kurup HV, Clark CIM, Dega RK. Footwear and orthopaedics. Foot Ankle Surg 2012;18:79–83.
18. Morio C, Lake MJ, Geuguen N, et al. The influence of footwear on motion during walking and running. J Biomech 2009;42:2081–8.
19. Thompson AT, Zipfel B, Muzigaba M, et al. Flexion location of the first metatarsalphalangeal joint and the location of forefoot ben in general purpose women's footwear. Foot Ankle Surg 2019;25(3):340–7.
20. Franklin S, Greay MJ, Heneghan N, et al. Barefoot vs common footwear: a systematic review of the kinematic, kinetic and muscle activity differences during walking. Gait Posture 2015;42:230–9.
21. Zhang X, Paquette MR, Zhang S. A comparison of gait biomechanics of flip flops, sandals, barefoot and shoes. J Foot Ankle Res 2013;45(6):45.
22. Nigg B, Hintzen S, Ferber R. Effect of unstable shoe construction on lower extremity gait characteristics. Clin Biomech 2006;21:82–8.
23. Khoury M, Wolf A, Debbi E, et al. Foot center of pressure trajectory alteration by biomechanical manipulation of shoe design. Foot Ankle Int 2013;34(4):593–8.

Surgical Biomechanics
Principles of Procedure Choice

Jarrod Shapiro, DPM

KEYWORDS

- Surgical biomechanics • Kineticokinematic approach • Kinetics • Kinematics
- Decision making

KEY POINTS

- Current research regarding the decision-making tree for surgical procedure choice is limited, especially in reference to kinetic data.
- A paucity of literature exists linking biomechanical changes with quality of life.
- Additionally, the majority of kinetic research is cadaveric, and extrapolation from the literature must be done with caution.
- An improved understanding of the kinetic and kinematic contributions to disease will allow surgeons to choose procedures and help guide future research.

INTRODUCTION

For many pathologic entities of the lower extremity, surgery is considered the treatment of last resort. Health care providers attempt to resolve painful conditions through various nonsurgical approaches, many of which utilize biomechanical principles.

When nonsurgical treatments fail to resolve patients' symptoms, surgery becomes the method of choice. A rich history of various surgical approaches to pathology of the lower extremity exists, ranging from soft tissue primary repair and augmentation to bone and joint osteotomy and/or arthrodesis procedures. When considering the thought process to choosing surgical procedures versus that of nonsurgical methods, however, there is a large discrepancy in methodology. The general inclination when treating patients clinically is to focus on the cause of the disease, understand its pathogenesis, and direct a treatment against that pathogenesis. An example of this is treatment of rheumatologic conditions, such as rheumatoid arthritis, with disease-modifying antirheumatic drugs or isolated joint injections with corticosteroids.

No commercial or financial conflicts of interest and no funding sources.
Western University of Health Sciences, College of Podiatric Medicine, Department of Podiatric Medicine, Surgery and Biomechanics, Chino Valley Medical Center Podiatric Medicine and Surgery Residency with Rearfoot Reconstruction and Ankle Certificate, 795 East 2nd Street, Suite 7, Pomona, CA 91766, USA
E-mail address: jshapiro@westernu.edu

Clin Podiatr Med Surg 37 (2020) 101–116
https://doi.org/10.1016/j.cpm.2019.08.009
0891-8422/20/© 2019 Elsevier Inc. All rights reserved.

podiatric.theclinics.com

On the contrary, when surgery is undertaken, the tendency has been to search for deformities and repair those deformities. The treatment of posterior tibial tendon dysfunction/adult-acquired flatfoot, for example, has historically focused on obtaining radiographs, measuring angles and relationships, and then choosing procedures to normalize those angles and relationships (with or without direct repair of the tendon). This endeavor has occurred with the assumption that postoperative normal radiographic appearance correlates positively with improved patient outcomes.[1,2] It is understandable that this approach is popular due to the availability of imaging modalities, ease of research methodology, and rarity and expense of biomechanical research equipment.

Despite these challenges, a measured approach to surgical decision making is necessary to choose the most appropriate procedures and obtain the best outcomes for patients. To that end, the purpose of this article is to describe the biomechanical background underlying surgical decision making and describe a unified approach to surgical procedure choice and discusses case examples that demonstrate the utility of this approach.

KINEMATIC BIOMECHANICAL PRINCIPLES

Surgical procedure choice may be considered via 1 of 2 primary perspectives: kinematics and kinetics. Defining these terms is instructive and allows for a more detailed consideration. Kinematics is the branch of mechanics concerned with the movement of objects (in this case, bones, joints, and soft tissue structures) without regard to the forces acting on them.[3] Kinetics focuses on the forces acting on structures that create movement rather than the positions of those structures.[4]

The biomechanics paradigm advocated by Root and colleagues[5] and adopted by most podiatrists is principally a kinematic one in which the clinician attempts to maintain the foot in a neutral subtalar joint position and to accommodate deformities to prevent compensation that lead to symptoms.

Similarly, the concept of planal dominance, originally conceived by Green and Carol[6] and adapted to surgery by many, including Borrelli and Smith,[7] is kinematic in emphasis. Borrelli and Smith clearly state, "Correction should always be directed to the area of deformity."[7] This view emphasizes relocating structures that are in an incorrect position back to a corrected or normal position. Because the lower extremity is a highly complex and variable machine, however, it often is difficult to determine what normal actually is.

Root and colleagues[5] attempted to standardize a definition of normal via the "biophysical criteria of normalcy" (**Box 1**). This set of characteristics may be better thought

---

Box 1
Root and colleagues' biophysical criteria of normalcy

- Distal one-third leg is vertical
- Posterior calcaneal bisection vertical
- Knee, ankle, subtalar joint parallel with floor (in transverse plane)
- Plantar forefoot parallels plantar rearfoot, both parallel with ground
- Metatarsals 2, 3, and 4 dorsiflexed position, all parallel with ground
- Metatarsal heads 1 and 5 in same plane as heads of 2, 3, and 4

Data from Root ML, et al. Biomechanical Examination of the Foot. Volume 1. 1971.

of as components of an ideal foot structure that a surgeon may aim for when choosing procedures. Contemporary research has not borne out these characteristics as common in the human population, and no research has validated this description. McPoil and colleagues[8] found a variety of foot positions in a group of 116 feet, with only 17% of patients fitting Root's normal criteria, whereas Garbalosa and colleagues'[9] measurement of 234 feet revealed forefoot varus positioning in 86.67% of the population and a perpendicular forefoot to rearfoot position in only 4.56%. The utility of an approach that focuses solely on position must be questioned (see **Box 1**).

The kinematic approach has been further utilized when creating radiographic parameters to aid in surgical evaluation and planning. Several investigators have described and tabulated various angles and relationships to qualify and quantify deformities.[6,10,11] An example of this is using the first intermetatarsal angle on dorsoplantar weight bearing radiographs to choose a bunionectomy procedure.[6] Labovitz[12] combined the planal dominance concept with radiographic angles to assist surgeons with procedure choice in approaching pediatric flatfoot deformities. Similarly, the determination of outcomes related to pes cavus reconstructive surgery is often quantified using Meary's angle.[13,14]

This position-related paradigm has most recently culminated in the center of rational angulation (CORA) concept and the delineation of osteotomy rules by Paley.[15] Using this paradigm, the surgeon, predominantly using standing full-limb radiographs, determines various axes of bones and positions of joints. Deviations from normal (malalignments of mechanical and anatomic axes) and the principle location of a deformity, the CORA, are calculated, and surgical procedures are aimed at correcting those malalignments.[16] This kinematic approach is well coupled with external fixation modalities[17] and provides a simple and quantifiable way to treat patients.

Improved outcomes for a large number of pathologic entities affecting the foot and ankle have been demonstrated reporting kinematic outcomes[1,2,18] and should not be discounted. It is also imperative, however, to understand that changing the position of bones and joints also have effects on pressure and force redistribution, and these changes may be the unrecognized cause of the reported improved outcomes. It is also important, however, to recognize that inappropriate procedure choice or failed appropriate procedures may increase deformity or create additional pathology.

KINETICS-ORIENTED BIOMECHANICS

Contemporary research has led to new biomechanical paradigms that focus on kinetics with the most visible being the subtalar axis location and rotational equilibrium theory, espoused by Kirby[19–21] (discussed later). In this theory, the transverse plane location of the subtalar joint axis is pivotal to foot function. If the subtalar joint is located too far medially, then ground reactive forces will be greater lateral to the subtalar axis, leading to increased pronation and the symptoms noted in patients with pronatory complaints. The converse is true with a subtalar axis located medial to the subtalar joint.

This approach has ramifications beyond axis location. The location of the subtalar axis additionally dictates the manner in which muscle-tendon units function on the foot.[20] Again, in the case of a medially deviated subtalar joint, tendons normally located medially then insert laterally, leading to subtalar pronation coupled with the normal action of the tendon. The Achilles tendon, for example, normally inserting medial to the subtalar joint axis, inserts lateral to the axis when it is pathologically medially deviated. This leads to subtalar joint pronation with ankle joint plantarflexion. Importantly, this system focuses not on position or kinematics but rather kinetics (forces acting on the foot).

Mueller and Maulf[22] discussed physical stress theory, commonly used in the physical therapy community, which has been adapted in the lower extremity as tissue stress theory.[23] The basic premise of this concept is that changes in physical stress cause predictable adaptive responses in tissue. This theory pays close attention to the stress placed on anatomic structures, which couples well with other kinetic theories. The major principles of this theory are described in **Box 2**.

McPoil and colleagues[23] adapted this model to create a 4-step approach to patient issues:

Step 1: determine specific injured anatomy.
Step 2: identify force-causing stress.
Step 3: determine structural or functional characteristics causing stress.
Step 4: design a plan.

This approach is primarily kinetic and focuses less on position being the cause of pathology; instead it emphasizes general characteristics surrounding the problem.

A UNIFIED APPROACH TO SURGICAL PROCEDURE CHOICE

The previous discussion leads to the conclusion that prior models of surgical procedure choice have been principally of kinematic type, whereas newer biomechanical

---

Box 2
Major principles of physical stress theory

1. Changes in relative level of physical stress cause predictable responses.

2. Five characteristic responses to stress: death, injury, increased tolerance (hypertrophy), maintenance, decreased tolerance (atrophy)

3. Physical stress levels lower than maintenance range result in decreased tolerance of tissues to subsequent stresses (atrophy).

4. Physical stress levels within the maintenance range result in no tissue damage.

5. Physical stress levels that exceed the maintenance range (overload) result in increased tolerance of tissues to subsequent stresses (hypertrophy).

6. Excessively high levels of physical stress result in tissue injury.

7. Extreme deviations from the maintenance stress that exceed the adaptive capacity of tissues result in tissue death.

8. Level of exposure to stress is a composite value defined by magnitude, time, and direction of stress.

9. Individual stresses combine in complex ways to contribute to the overall level of stress. Tissues are affected by the history of recent stress.

10. Injury can occur by
    A. High stress over a brief period
    B. Low stress over a long period
    C. Moderate stress applied many times

11. Inflammation occurs immediately after tissue injury, rendering the tissue less tolerant of stress. Must protect inflamed tissues from subsequent excessive stress until inflammation resolves.

12. Stress thresholds vary among patients, depending on several modulating factors, including movement, alignment, extrinsic, behavioral, and physiologic factors.

Data from Mueller M, Maulf K. Tissue Adaptation to Physical Stress: A Proposed "Physical Stress Theory" to Guide Physical Therapist Practice, Education, and Research. Physical Therapy, Apr 2002; 82(4): 383 - 403.

frameworks have increasingly focused on kinetics. Instead of separating the 2, the author advocates a different paradigm, which is a patient outcome–centered rather than position-centered approach. This method of surgical procedure choice incorporates a combined kinematic and kinetic approach, termed the kineticokinematic (KK) approach, described in **Box 3**.

Using this decision-making paradigm creates a systematic approach that incorporates current biomechanical models while maintaining the success of prior approaches. It also focuses on the anatomic damage with increased focus on the cause.

Step 1: Determine the Strained or Damaged Anatomic Structure(s)

The KK approach begins with a full and complete history and physical examination of the patient with the goal of determining which anatomic structure or structures are involved. In cases of lower extremity ulcerations (**Figs. 1** and **2**), it is rapidly apparent what is damaged. In other situations, such as plantar fasciitis, palpation easily determines the affected pathoanatomy.

In other situations, such as posterior tibial tendon dysfunction/adult acquired flatfoot deformity, a more thorough search for involved anatomy must be undertaken. Examination of the posterior tibial tendon for insertional versus tendon body pain, stability of the spring ligament complex,[24] single-limb heel rise, and individual muscle strength testing help determine the specific pathoanatomy and rules out involvement of other tissues.

Step 2: Clarify the Underlying Biomechanical Cause of the Strained Anatomy

Once the provider determines which structures are damaged, the cause of the strain, stress, or damage is elucidated. This is attained by understanding the pathomechanics and forces acting on the lower extremity and is accomplished via completion of the physical examination coupled with a detailed understanding of biomechanics of the lower extremity.

For example, plantar fasciitis has been determined to be a disorder of myxoid collagen degeneration, marrow vascular dilation, and a lack of inflammatory changes on tissue pathology.[25] Additionally, a greater magnitude of rearfoot eversion, medial forefoot dorsiflexion,[26] and equinus[27] have been found in patients with a diagnosis of plantar fasciitis. An understanding of these mechanical contributions may be helpful in choosing surgical procedures. This explains why the addition of a gastrocnemius recession procedure has been shown to improve symptoms in patients with plantar fasciitis[27,28] (**Fig. 3**).

An improved appreciation of the biomechanics literature may also improve understanding of the effects surgical procedures have on the foot. The Lapidus procedure, for example, although initially described for the correction of hallux valgus deformity, has been found to have additional effects on the foot. Roling and colleagues[29] found

---

Box 3
A unified kinetokinematic paradigm for surgical procedure choice providing a stepwise approach for patient evaluation and surgical thought process

KK approach to surgical procedure choice

1. Determine the damaged anatomic structure under stress.

2. Clarify the underlying biomechanical cause of the strain.

3. Revise the pathomechanical issue by adjusting internal forces and/or correcting deformity.

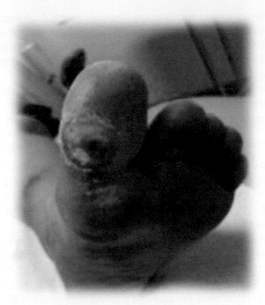

Fig. 1. Classic neuropathic ulceration in a diabetic patient where the damaged anatomy is clear.

medial column motion to be distributed across the 3 joints of the arch with first metatarsocuneiform motion 41%, naviculocuneiform motion 50%, and talonavicular joint motion 9% of total arch motion. Perez and colleagues[30] expanded on this with the physical confirmation of the first metatarsocuneiform joint to be important to motion of the medial column. When the first metatarsal is in an everted position, the joint

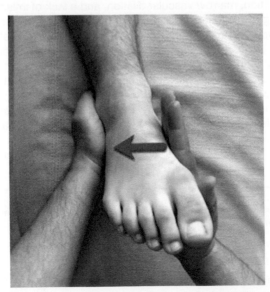

Fig. 2. The neutral heel, lateral push test to determine integrity of the spring ligament complex. Arrow indicates lateral direction of force in which right hand is pushing.

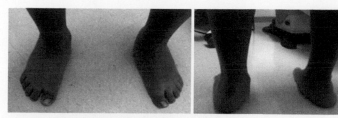

Fig. 3. Subtalar pronation in a patient with plantar fascia insertional pain as evidenced by the everted resting calcaneal stance position (right image) and plantarmedially prominent talar head (left and right images). Appreciating these accessory deformities assists the provider with understanding the etiology of the damaged tissue.

achieves a close-packed confirmation with improved arch stability. Coupling this information with the known function of the peroneus longus tendon as an everter of the first metatarsal[31] creates a powerful biomechanical explanation for the arch stabilizing effect of the Lapidus procedure and elects it as an appropriate candidate procedure for flatfoot reconstruction.

Understanding the forces acting on the foot is also necessary to clarify the biomechanics of the abnormal foot. At this time, it is difficult for the average foot and ankle surgeon to obtain direct information about pedal force and pressure distribution due to the cost of technology. Some available measurement technology is discussed elsewhere in this issue. It thus becomes necessary to rely on indirect physical examination techniques, such as identification of hyperkeratotic lesions, and research literature to identify the forces acting on the foot.

Kirby[21] has described a simple and reproducible examination technique to determine the transverse plane location of the subtalar joint axis. This method (**Fig. 4**) allows the surgeon to locate the axis and extrapolate ground reactive forces pushing dorsally on the foot relative to that axis, causing subtalar pronation (in a medially deviated axis) (**Fig. 5**) and supination (in a laterally deviated axis). This technique has been validated to have good to excellent intrarater reliability of 0.78 to 0.95 and inter-rater reliability of 0.72 to 0.96.[32]

Step 3: Correct the Underlying Abnormal Biomechanics and Strain by Adjusting the Forces that Act on the Lower Extremity and/or Realigning Deformity

The surgeon executes a surgical plan by choosing procedures that counter abnormal biomechanical function, thereby adjusting abnormal forces to establish normal function. This may or may not include correction of deformity itself and is unconcerned with restoration of strict radiographic parameters. It becomes important for surgeons to understand the biomechanical effects of specific surgical procedures in order to choose appropriate surgeries. To aid in understanding the mechanical effects of surgical procedures on the foot and ankle, **Table 1** lists the consequences of common osteotomies, arthrodesis, and other surgeries.

Use of the KK approach to choosing surgical procedures can be further elucidated through specific case examples.

CASE 1: NEUROPATHIC ULCER IN A DIABETIC PATIENT WITH PES CAVUS

Patient DM was a 52-year-old type 2 diabetic man with a neuropathic ulceration plantar to the tibial sesamoid. A prior tibial sesamoidectomy was performed, but the patient continued to ulcerate despite total contact cast offloading, moist wound

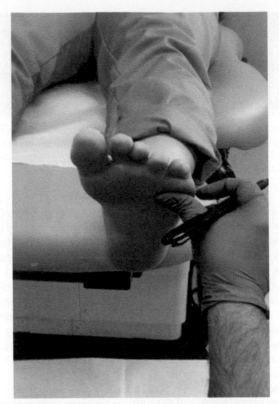

Fig. 4. Representation of identifying the location of the subtalar joint axis using the concept of rotational equilibrium.

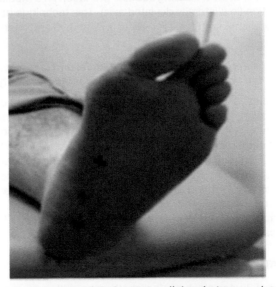

Fig. 5. Physical examination using the plantar parallel technique to determine a medially deviated subtalar joint axis, allowing an appreciation of the pronatory ground reactive forces acting on the foot.

Table 1
Selected common reconstructive foot and ankle surgical procedures and associated kinetic and kinematic effects

Procedure	Kinematic Effects	Kinetic Effects
Osteotomies		
Evans calcaneal osteotomy	Establishment of improved peroneus longus tendon function with first ray plantarflexion[31]	• Decreased first metatarsal load[33] • Decreased talonavicular joint moment[33] • Increased lateral column load[33,34]
Medial displacement calcaneal osteotomy	• Medialization of the Achilles tendon[35] • Axial relocation of the calcaneus under the tibia (realigning the mechanical axis of the limb)[36]	• Decreased first metatarsal load[37] • Decreased talonavicular joint moment[37] • Increased lateral column load[37] • 1 cm medial displacement moves tibiotalar center of pressure 1.0–1.58 mm medially[36,38]
Dwyer calcaneal osteotomy	• 7–8 mm available lateralizing, 18.2 mm of lateralization with the classic osteotomy[39,40] • Greater correction possible with wedge resection[39] • 3 mm lateralization of Achilles[40] • Improved lateralization of heel with slide added to Dwyer[41]	Unknown
Lateral displacement calcaneal osteotomy	• 12.7 mm available lateralizing[39] • Greater correction possible with wedge resection[39]	1 cm lateral displacement moves tibiotalar center of pressure 1-mm laterally[36,38]
Cotton osteotomy	Correction of forefoot varus position[a]	Unknown
Arthrodeses		

Medial column arthrodeses	• First metatarsocuneiform
	  ○ 41% reduced medial column motion (Roling)
	  ○ Increased frontal plane eversion, talar dorsiflexion[42]
	• Naviculocuneiform—50% reduced medial column motion[29]
	• Talonavicular—9% reduced medial column motion[29]
		First metatarsocuneiform
		  ○ Decreased hallux plantar pressure[43]
		  ○ Decreased plantar second metatarsal head pressure[43]
		  ○ Increased fifth metatarsal head plantar pressure[43]

Hindfoot arthrodeses	• Subtalar—26% talonavicular joint motion remained; 56% calcaneocuboid joint motion remained[44] • Talonavicular—limited hindfoot motion to 2°, limited posterior tibial tendon excursion to 25% of original value[44] • Calcaneocuboid—limited talonavicular joint motion by 33%, limited subtalar joint motion by 8%[44] • Similar findings by Wülker[45]	Subtalar, double, triple arthrodeses—decreased ankle contact force and contact area. Decreased peak contact stress when rectus or everted and increased when inverted.[46]

(continued on next page)

Table 1 (continued)		
Procedure	**Kinematic Effects**	**Kinetic Effects**
Ankle arthrodesis	• Decreased cadence and stride length[47] • Decreased hindfoot and midfoot motion all planes during gait[47,48]	• Increased talonavicular joint and calcaneocuboid joint pressure on inclines[49] • Increased midfoot stress[50] • Earlier anterior movement of ground reaction force in early gait[50]
Soft tissue procedures		
Gastrocnemius recession	• Increased ankle dorsiflexion[51] • No changes in gait kinetics or kinematics[52]	• Reduced forefoot peak plantar pressures[53] • No changes to ankle or knee mechanics[52]
Achilles tendon lengthening	Increased ankle dorsiflexion	Reduced forefoot peak plantar pressures[54]
Other		
Subtalar arthroeiresis	Improved radiographic parameters (Meary's, talar covering, forefoot adduction)[18]	• Decreased load on medial arch[55] • Decreased talonavicular joint moment[55]

[a] No research evidence to confirm effect.

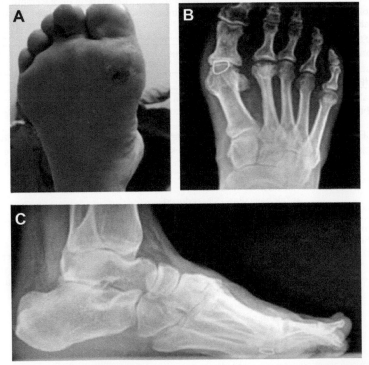

Fig. 6. (*A*) Preoperative clinical and (*B*) radiographic images of a diabetic patient with a recurrent subtibial sesamoid ulceration despite sesamoidectomy. (*C*) Lateral view of radiographic image. Note the lesion marker showing the ulcer location just distal to the prior tibial sesamoid.

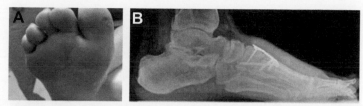

Fig. 7. (*A*) Clinical and (*B*) lateral radiographic images status post–dorsiflexory first metatar-socuneiform arthrodesis, first metatarsophalangeal joint arthroplasty with synthetic carti-lage implant, and gastrocnemius recession demonstrating complete healing without recurrence.

care, and débridement (**Fig. 6**A). Preoperative radiographs with a lesion marker at the ulcer site demonstrated the location to be just distal to the previously removed sesa-moid and confirmation of an anterior lesser tarsus pes cavus foot type with apex at the tarsometatarsal joint (**Fig. 6**B, C).

Utilizing the KK approach, step 1 showed the tissue under stress was the plantar first metatarsal head tissue. Step 2 of the KK algorithm included a full examination, which revealed the following pertinent findings: a pes cavus foot type, forefoot valgus with rigidly plantarflexed first metatarsal, hallux rigidus with no more than 10° of dorsi-flexion, and decreased ankle joint dorsiflexion with the knee flexed that improved past neutral with the knee flexed.

It was clear that procedure choice, utilizing the KK approach, conceptually required decreasing peak plantar forefoot pressures. This thought process led to a dorsiflexory first metatarsocuneiform arthrodesis, first metatarsophalangeal joint arthroplasty with synthetic cartilage implant, and gastrocnemius recession. These procedures success-fully resolved the ulceration without recurrence by not only improving the cavus defor-mity (kinematic change) but also decreasing plantar forefoot pressures (kinetic change) (**Fig. 7**).

CASE 2: POSTERIOR TIBIAL TENDON DYSFUNCTION/ADULT ACQUIRED FLATFOOT

Patient CD was a 46-year-old woman complaining of a painful medial ankle with a his-tory consistent with posterior tibial tendon dysfunction. Examination revealed pain to palpation along the body of the posterior tibial tendon, without insertional pain, an inability to perform the single-limb heel rise, pain and abduction with the neutral heel lateral push test, and fully flexible medial arch excursion. A gastrocnemius equi-nus also was measured. Standing and gait examination (**Fig. 8**A, B) indicated a rectus

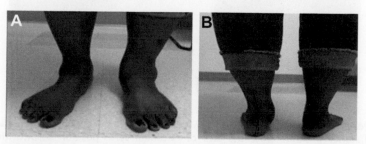

Fig. 8. Preoperative clinical appearance with focus on the right lower extremity. (*A*) Front view and (*B*) back view.

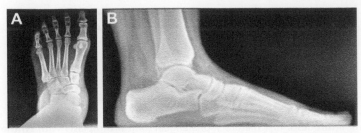

Fig. 9. Preoperative radiographs demonstrating a primarily transverse plane dominant flat-foot deformity evidenced by talar head uncovering and increased calcaneocuboid abduction angle (calcaneal axial radiographs not available). (*A*) Top view and (*B*) lateral view.

heel, forefoot abduction, and lack of resupination during the late stance phase of gait. Radiographs are shown in **Fig. 9**A, B.

The KK approach first defines this patient's strained and contributing anatomy primarily as the posterior tibial tendon and spring ligament complex. The underlying biomechanical issues were determined to be a medially deviated subtalar joint axis, excessive pronation, and high medial arch strain forces, which led to overloaded medial support structures and posterior tibial tendon strain.

As a result of these considerations, surgical procedure choice included the following: medial displacement calcaneal osteotomy to decrease medial arch strain,[37] Evans osteotomy to adduct the forefoot and reestablish peroneus longus tendon function for improved arch supination (resulting from retrograde pull from a close-packed first metatarsocuneiform joint), and allograft spring ligament reconstruction with interference screw fixation based on the importance of the spring ligament as the primary arch-supporting structure.[56] A gastrocnemius recession was not performed. By medializing the calcaneus in relation to the subtalar axis, a longer Achilles lever arm was created, increasing the supinatory power of the gastrocnemius soleus complex.[35]

Postoperatively, the patient had improved kinematic parameters with decreased talar adduction (**Fig. 10**A) and rectus resting calcaneal stance position (**Fig. 10**B).

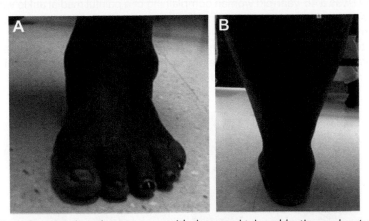

Fig. 10. Postoperative clinical appearance with decreased talar adduction and rectus resting calcaneal stance position. Note the lack of calcaneal varus position despite the medial displacement on a previously rectus preoperative heel position. (*A*) Front view and (*B*) back view.

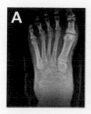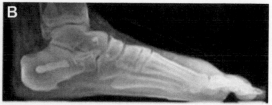

Fig. 11. Postoperative radiographic appearance demonstrating normalization of kinematic parameters. (A) Top view and (B) lateral view.

Radiographically, the calcaneal inclination angle improved in addition to complete talar head covering and rectus calcaneocuboid joint alignment, indicating a triplanar correction. No medial column arthrodeses were performed, and all kinematic parameters were improved without resorting to fusions.

Because there are few available clinical methods to measure postoperative kinetic results, it must be extrapolated that this patient had improved kinetics from the complete resolution of posterior tibial tendon pain (see **Figs. 8–10; Fig. 11**).

FUTURE DIRECTIONS

Current research regarding the decision-making tree for surgical procedure choice is limited, especially in reference to kinetic data. A paucity of literature exists linking biomechanical changes with quality of life. Additionally, the majority of kinetic research is cadaveric, and extrapolation from the literature must be done with caution.

Future research should increasingly focus not only on all aspects of surgical procedures, both kinetics and kinematics, but also on patient quality of life and cost effectiveness. Finally, there is a strong need for new technologies to better study kinetics in vivo. With these issues resolved, the ability of surgeons to rationally choose and execute procedures will move the profession forward for the benefit of patients.

REFERENCES

1. Lee MS, Vanore JV, Thomas JL, et al. Clinical practice guideline: diagnosis and treatment of adult flatfoot. J Foot Ankle Surg 2005;44(2):79–113.
2. Catanzariti AR, Lee MS, Mendicino RW. Posterior calcaneal displacement osteotomy for adult acquired flatfoot. J Foot Ankle Surg 2000;39(1):2–14.
3. Merriam-webster online dictionary. Available at. www.merriam-webster.com/dictionary/kinematics. Accessed May 9, 2019.
4. Merriam-webster online dictionary. Available at. www.merriam-webster.com/dictionary/kinetics. Accessed May 9, 2019.
5. Root ML, Orien WP, Weed JH, et al. Biomechanical examination of the foot, volume 1. Los Angeles: Clinical Biomechanics Corporation; 1971. p. 34.
6. Green DR, Carol A. Planal dominance. J Am Podiatr Med Assoc 1984;74(2):98–103.
7. Borrelli A, Smith S. Surgical considerations in the treatment of pes planus. J Am Podiatr Med Assoc 1988;78(6):305–9.
8. McPoil TG, Knecht HG, Schuit D. A survey of foot types in normal females between the ages of 18 and 30 years. J Orthop Sports Phys Ther 1988;9(12):406–9.
9. Garbalosa JC, McClure MH, Catlin PA, et al. The frontal plane relationship of the forefoot to the rearfoot in n asymptomatic population. J Orthop Sports Phys Ther 1994;20(4):200–6.

10. Lamm BM, Stasko PA, Gesheff MG, et al. Normal foot and ankle radiographic angles, measurements, and reference points. J Foot Ankle Surg 2016;55:991–8.
11. Green DR. Radiology and biomechanical foot types. Surgery of the foot and leg update. Tucker (GA): The Podiatry Institute; 1998.
12. Labovitz J. The algorithmic approach to pediatric flexible pes planovalgus. Clin Podiatr Med Surg 2006;23(1):57–76.
13. Johnson BM, Child B, Hix J, et al. Cavus foot reconstruction in 3 patients with charcot-marie-tooth disease. J Foot Ankle Surg 2009;48(2):116–24.
14. Boffeli T, Collier R. Surgical technique for combined dwyer calcaneal osteotomy and peroneal tendon repair for correction of peroneal tendon pathology associated with cavus foot deformity. J Foot Ankle Surg 2012;51:135–40.
15. Paley D. Principles of deformity correction. Berlin: Springer-Verlag; 2003.
16. Lamm B, Paley D. Deformity correction planning for hindfoot, ankle, and lower limb. Clin Podiatr Med Surg 2004;21(3):305–26.
17. Paley D, Tetsworth K. Deformity correction by the ilizarov technique. Operative orthopaedics. 2nd edition. Philadelphia: B. Lippincott Company; 1993.
18. Walley KC, Greene G, Hallam J, et al. Short- to mid-term outcomes following the use of an arthroeresis implant as an adjunct for correction of flexible, acquired flatfoot deformity in adults. Foot Ankle Spec 2018;12(2):122–30.
19. Kirby K. Rotational equilibrium across the subtalar joint axis. J Am Podiatr Med Assoc 1989;79(1):1–13.
20. Kirby K. Subtalar joint axis location and rotational equilibrium theory of foot function. J Am Podiatr Med Assoc 2001;91(9):465–87.
21. Kirby K. Methods for determination of positional variations in the subtalar joint axis. J Am Podiatr Med Assoc 1987;77(5):228–34.
22. Mueller M, Maulf K. Tissue adaptation to physical stress: a proposed "physical stress theory" to guide physical therapist practice, education, and research. Phys Ther 2002;82(4):383–403.
23. McPoil TG, Hunt GC. Evaluation and management of foot and ankle disorders: present problems and future directions. J Orthop Sports Phys Ther 1995;21(6):381–8.
24. Pasapula C, Devany A, Magan A, et al. Neutral heel lateral push test: the first clinical examination of spring ligament integrity. Foot (Edinb) 2015;25(2):69–74.
25. Lemont H, Ammirati KM, Usen N. Plantar fasciitis: a degenerative process (Fasciosis) without inflammation. J Am Podiatr Med Assoc 2003;93(3):234–7.
26. Riddle DL, Pulisic M, Pidcoe P, et al. Risk factors for plantar fasciitis: a matched case-control study. J Bone Joint Surg 2003;85-A(5):872–7.
27. Chang R, Rodrigues PA, Van Emmerik RE, et al. Multi-segment foot kinematics and ground reaction forces during gait of individuals with plantar fasciitis. J Biomech 2014;47:2571–7.
28. Monteagudo M, Maceira E, Garcia-Virto V, et al. Chronic plantar fasciitis: plantar fasciotomy versus gastrocnemius recession. Int Orthop 2013;37:1845–50.
29. Roling BA, Christensen JC, Johnson CH. Biomechanics of the first ray. Part IV: the effect of selected medial column arthrodeses a three-dimensional kinematic analysis in a cadaver model. J Foot Ankle Surg 2002;41(5):278–85.
30. Perez HR, Reber LK, Christensen JC. The effect of frontal plane position on first ray motion: forefoot lockingmechanism. Foot Ankle Int 2008;29(1):72–6.
31. Johnson C, Christensen J. Biomechanics of the first ray. Part I. The effects of peroneus longus function: a three-dimensional kinematic study on a cadaver model. J Foot Ankle Surg 1999;38(5):313–21.

32. Van Alsenoy K, D'Août K, Vereecke EE, et al. The subtalar joint axis palpation technique part 2: reliability and validity results using cadaver feet. J Am Podiatr Med Assoc 2014;104(4):365–74.

33. Arangio GA, Chopra V, Voloshin A, et al. A biomechanical analysis of the effect of lateral column lengthening calcaneal osteotomy on the flat foot. Clin Biomech 2007;22:472–7.

34. Pratley EM, Matheis EA, Hayes CW, et al. Effects of degree of surgical correction for flatfoot deformity in patient-specific computational models. Ann Biomed Eng 2015;43(8):1947–56.

35. Sung IH, Lee S, Otis JC, et al. Posterior tibial tendon force requirement in early heel rise after calcaneal osteotomies. Foot Ankle Int 2002;23(9):842–9.

36. Steffensmeier SJ, Berbaum KS, Brown TD. Effects of medial and lateral displacement calcaneal osteotomies on tibiotalar joint contact stresses. J Orthop Res 1996;14(6):980–5.

37. Arangio G, Salathe E. A biomechanical analysis of posterior tibial tendon dysfunction, medial displacement calcaneal osteotomy and flexor digitorum longus transfer in adult acquired flat foot. Clin Biomech 2009;24:385–90.

38. Davitt JS, Beals TC, Bachus KN. The effects of medial and lateral displacement calcaneal osteotomies on ankle and subtalar joint pressure distribution. Foot Ankle Int 2001;22(11):885–9.

39. Cody EA, Kraszewski AP, Conti MS, et al. Lateralizing calcaneal osteotomies and their effect on calcaneal alignment: a three-dimensional digital model analysis. Foot Ankle Int 2018;39(8):970–7.

40. An TW, Michalski M, Jansson K, et al. Comparison of lateralizing calcaneal osteotomies for varus hindfoot correction. Foot Ankle Int 2018;39(10):1229–36.

41. Pfeffer GB, Michalski MP, Basak T, et al. Use of 3D prints to compare the efficacy of three different calcaneal osteotomies for the correction of heel varus. Foot Ankle Int 2018;39(5):591–7.

42. King CM, Hamilton GA, Ford LA. Effects of the lapidus arthrodesis and chevron bunionectomy on plantar forefoot pressures. J Foot Ankle Surg 2014;53:415–9.

43. Bierman R, Christensen J, Johnson C. Biomechanics of the first ray part III. Consequences of lapidus arthrodesis on peroneus longus function: a three-dimensional kinematic study on a cadaver model. J Foot Ankle Surg 2001; 39(2):125–31.

44. Astion DJ, Deland JT, Otis JC, et al. Motion of the hindfoot after simulated arthrodesis. J Bone Joint Surg 1997;79-A(2):241–6.

45. Wülker N, Stukenborg C, Savory KM, et al. Hindfoot motion after isolated and combined arthrodeses: measurements in anatomic specimens. Foot Ankle Int 2000;21(11):921–7.

46. Hutchinson ID, Baxter JR, Gilbert S, et al. How do hindfoot fusions affect ankle biomechanics: a cadaver model. Clin Orthop Relat Res 2016;474(4):1008–16.

47. Thomas R, Daniels TR, Parker K. Gait analysis and functional outcomes following ankle arthrodesis for isolated ankle arthritis. J Bone Joint Surg Am 2006;88(3): 526–35.

48. Valderrabano V, Hintermann B, Nigg BM, et al. Kinematic changes after fusion and total replacement of the ankle: part 2: movement transfer. Foot Ankle Int 2003;24(12):888–96.

49. Jung HG, Parks BG, Nguyen A, et al. Effect of tibiotalar joint arthrodesis on adjacent tarsal joint pressure in a cadaver model. Foot Ankle Int 2007;28(1):103–8.

50. Beyaert C, Sirveaux F, Paysant J, et al. The effect of tibio-talar arthrodesis on foot kinematics and ground reaction force progression during walking. Gait Posture 2004;20(1):84–91.
51. Gianakos A, Yasui Y, Murawski CD, et al. Effects of gastrocnemius recession on ankle motion, strength, and functional outcomes: a systematic review and national healthcare database analysis. Knee Surg Sports Traumatol Arthrosc 2016;24:1355–64.
52. Chimera NJ, Castro M, Davis I, et al. The effect of isolated gastrocnemius contracture and gastrocnemius recession on lower extremity kinematics and kinetics during stance. Clin Biomech 2012;27:917–23.
53. Greenhagen RM, Johnson AR, Peterson MC, et al. Gastrocnemius recession as an alternative to tendoachilles lengthening for relief of forefoot pressure in a patient with peripheral neuropathy: a case report and description of a technical modification. J Foot Ankle Surg 2010;49(2):159.e9-13.
54. Armstrong DG, Stacpoole-Shea S, Nguyen H, et al. Lengthening of the achilles tendon in diabetic patients who are at high risk for ulceration of the foot. J Bone Joint Surg 1999;81-A(4):535–8.
55. Arangio GA, Reinert KL, Salathe EP. A biomechanical model of the effect of subtalar arthreiresis on the adult flexible flat foot. Clin Biomech 2004;19:847–52.
56. Jennings M, Christensen J. The effects of sectioning the spring ligament on rearfoot stability and posterior tibial tendon efficiency. J Foot Ankle Surg 2008;47(3): 219–24.

Biomechanical Considerations in Rearfoot Fusions

Harold D. Schoenhaus, DPM[a,b,]*

KEYWORDS

- Biomechanics of foot and ankle • Rearfoot fusions • Total ankle joint replacements
- Triple arthrodesis • Phasic activity of muscles

KEY POINTS

- Understanding normal foot function is essential in presurgical planning. A rationale must be determined to enhance the outcome of the procedure and enable a thorough discussion with the patient so an informed decision can be made.
- When advanced procedures are determined, the ultimate effect on position and function will be established. The complexity of the foot secondary to triplane function and joint interactions demands a level of expertise to avoid predetermined complications.
- The direct correlation of ankle, subtalar, and midtarsal function is discussed. The comparison of open versus closed chain function is reviewed, including transverse plane motion of the leg with direct influence on the foot. The anatomy is reviewed in detail.

INTRODUCTION AND GENERAL MECHANICS

According to Inman,[1] the joints of the ankle should be considered to include the ankle, subtalar and midtarsal joints, recognizing their critical function relative to normal foot function. This definition could include the Lisfranc articulation as well because it is significantly affected by Charcot disease, with major destruction and alteration of normal foot function.[2–4]

There are many factors influencing normal function, such as trauma, single-plane osseous deformities, equinus, and congenital abnormalities. In addition, congenital clubbed foot, neurologic disorders, and Charcot-Marie-Tooth disease, along with degenerative arthritis and neuropathy, create associated motor dysfunction. Because the ankle, subtalar, and midtarsal joints are triplanar, they have the ability to compensate for deformity or deforming forces, which significant influences foot function.[5] Any

Disclosure: The author has nothing to disclose.
[a] Penn Presbyterian Medical Center, Philadelphia, PA, USA; [b] Temple University School of Podiatric Medicine, Philadelphia, PA, USA
* 16009 Brier Creek Drive, Delray Beach, FL 33446.
E-mail address: Podharold@gmail.com

Clin Podiatr Med Surg 37 (2020) 117–123
https://doi.org/10.1016/j.cpm.2019.08.010
0891-8422/20/© 2019 Elsevier Inc. All rights reserved.

compensatory mechanism influences function on the affected side as well as the contralateral side.[5]

According to Root and colleagues,[5] gait should be smooth and translatory with a minimal amount of energy expenditure. Lower extremity surgeons continually treat patients who develop symptoms secondary to these influences on normal function. During gait, axial rotation from the leg dominates and directs foot motion as ground reactive forces create a response, which is seen as pronatory and supinatory activity.[6] The subtalar joint acts as a torque converter, allowing the transitional force and position from heel strike to toe-off.[7,8] When abnormalities exist, the timing of transition is greatly affected, preventing relocation and stability into the propulsive phase of gait. An example of this adverse effect is hypermobility of the first ray with the development of hallux rigidus or hallux abductovalgus deformity. The author has attempted to treat these compensatory activities with orthotic control, providing reduction of symptoms and attempting to neutralize deforming forces.

This concept applies from pediatrics through to the geriatric population. When patients deviate from normal function, the phasic activity of extrinsic muscles of the leg, which show antagonistic, synergistic, or stabilizing activity, are also affected.[9] The resultant deformities, such as posterior tibial dysfunction, peroneal tears, hypermobility of the first ray, and Achilles disorders, are seen. A thorough knowledge of normal phasic activity is essential considering how many tendons are lengthened or transferred to alter function.[10] Determination of position and function becomes acutely critical in the diabetic population, because excessive pressure from abnormal position can lead to selected added pressure, ending in areas of tissue breakdown and ulceration.

ANKLE JOINT

The ankle joint is usually considered a ginglymus joint, with the dominant motion occurring in the sagittal plane.[5] Its axis of motion runs from the tip of the lateral malleolus up toward the tip of the medial malleolus. Furthermore, the anatomy of the joint is unique because of the shape of the talus and because it contains 3 different articular facets: medial, lateral, and dorsal. The talus is also tapered from anterior to posterior on its dorsal articulation. The posterior aspect is now lower than the distal portion, creating stability problems when the joint is plantarflexed. Strong lateral ligaments, such as the anterior talofibular, calcaneofibular, and posterior talofibular ligaments, add to the lateral stability of the ankle complex. The calcaneofibular ligament also provides additional stability to the subtalar joints. Medially, the deltoid complex is critical for stability, preventing pronatory forces, which would affect a total ankle joint replacement. The inferior tibiofibular syndesmotic ligament is essential to allow stability change as the foot moves in the sagittal plane. If there is posttraumatic injury to this ligament, widening of the mortise can occur, once again influencing the stability of a total ankle joint replacement.[11]

The foot (talus) is locked in the ankle mortise and responds differently with open versus closed kinetic chain movement. In open chain, the talus predominantly moves in the sagittal plane with minimal supinatory and pronatory affect. In closed chain motion, the axial rotation of the leg causes the talus to adduct and plantarflex, which causes the subtalar joint to pronate with direct influence on both axes of the midtarsal joint.[5] A reversal of this process occurs as the leg, during weight bearing, rotates and creates the reversal process of resupination. This process is the result of the contralateral limb going into toe-off.[12] In order for this process to occur, ankle stability is critical. The malleoli act as stirrups on the sides of the talus. However, trauma to ligaments or malleolar fractures can have adverse effects on normal function. In addition, tendon dysfunction, such as posterior tibial tendon disease or peroneal disorder, also influences ankle and foot function. In close chain motion, posterior tibial dysfunction causes excessive foot flattening, altering the ability of the subtalar and midtarsal joint to resupinate. This condition causes the ankle to respond to external rotation of the weight-bearing limb. The peroneals provide midstance and first-ray stability, allowing the transition of force to the forefoot for propulsive and first-ray stability.[13]

With the development of ankle joint replacement and multiple designs, manufacturers have not been able to determine why the complication rates are so high, as has been seen with the Agility ankle, even though numerous modifications have been made.[14] Ultimately it has led to it being removed from the marketplace. When degenerative joint disease of the ankle occurs, it is painful and excessive, usually secondary to trauma (fracture and sprains). The subtalar complex is usually affected as well. If the subtalar joint cannot function as a torque convertor, the transverse plane motion of the leg will influence the ankle, thus leading to abnormal polycomponent wear as well as subsidence and ectopic bone formation.[15] In theory, multiple-bearing ankle joints should alleviate some of these problems. If the subtalar joint is diseased, a fusion before or along with acute replacement is often recommended. This procedure accelerates abnormal forces at the ankle, leading to failure. Note that, if an ankle is fused, the loss of dorsiflexion is often compensated at the ball-and-socket talonavicular joint with minimal effect on foot function.[16,17] In addition, if the subtalar joint is relatively normal, protonation and supination can continue. This finding raises the question of fusion versus total ankle joint replacements in patients with degenerative joint disease of the ankle. Clinicians must also remember that the ankle joint is pronatory and supinatory. No implant accounts for this. In addition, deltoid insufficiency and frontal plane deformities must be considered and/or addressed when total ankle joint replacement is performed.[18]

SUBTALAR JOINT

The subtalar joint is 3 joints. The posterior facet, which is the largest, is separated from the anterior and middle facet by the sinus tarsi. The lateral part of the sinus tarsi contains a fibrofatty plug and the root is formed by the anterior talofibular ligament.[19] There is also the lateral ligament protecting the contents of the canal laterally. The medial portion of the sinus tarsi contains the interosseous talocalcaneal ligament, through which a neurovascular bundle is present. Proprioception of the subtalar position is monitored through this ligament. Ankle sprains often lead to sinus tarsitis; sinus tarsi syndrome/medial ligament dysfunction is associated with peritalar subluxation as well.[20] The anterior facet lies on the sustentaculum tali and is supported by the flexor hallucis longus tendon. During propulsion, the hallux dorsiflexes to 65°, increasing tension on the flexor hallucis longus and helping to provide supinatory forces on the subtalar joint.[5] The head of the talus sits on the anterior facet and is supported by the talocalcaneonavicular spring ligament. The middle facet helps support the lateral aspect of the talocalcaneal complex.[19]

The subtalar axis passes from posterior, inferior, and lateral to anterior, medial, and dorsal. Thus, the motion of this joint complex is triplanar. More specifically, pronatory-supinatory motion is appreciated at this joint complex. The axis deviates 16° from the sagittal plane; thus, it represents the least component of motion at the subtalar joint.[7,21]

The importance of this is that, to compensate for equinus, the subtalar joint must pronate excessively, primarily to unlock the midtarsal joint.[22] However, the longitudinal midtarsal axis is unlocked, leading to forefoot supinatus, a triplane soft tissue deformity.[23] It is critical to maintain subtalar position to provide stability to the midtarsal complex; thus, the concept of the rearfoot controlling the forefoot.[24] The bifurcate ligament helps to maintain proper position of the midtarsal joint and allows medial and lateral column function.[19] The lateral column is responsible for stability and the medial column mobility.[25]

As far as the subtalar joint is concerned, fusion may be necessary as an isolated procedure, after calcaneal factures, or secondary to tarsal coalitions.[26] Two important points must be considered. First, fusion directly affects ankle function because of loss of torque conversion capability, and degenerative joint disease of the ankle may develop with associated synovitis.[27] Second, the position of fusion is critical.[27] A slightly pronated position is far more acceptable for weight transfer to avoid lateral forefoot overload and potential secondary ankle sprains.[28,29] In addition, a supinated position allows an imbalance of power between the tibialis posterior and peroneus brevis, leading to a supinated position of the midtarsal joint.

Because the rearfoot controls the forefoot, this must be taken into account during fusion of the subtalar joint. This concept can also be appreciated with sinus tarsi implantation for flatfoot. Oversizing leads to overcorrection in a supinated position and is not compatible with normal function. In general, a slightly pronated foot is better functionally than a supinated position.[29]

THE MIDTARSAL JOINT

The midtarsal joint is 2 joints, providing pronatory and supinatory function. The calcaneocuboid joint is part of the lateral column of the foot and is the stable anatomic structure.[25] The talonavicular joint is considered part of the medial column of the foot and is considered dynamic. The shape of these two joints is significantly different, creating stability versus mobility. The calcaneocuboid joint is saddle shaped and is far more stable than the ball-and-socket talonavicular joint. The calcaneocuboid joint has dorsolateral and bifurcate ligament attachments, whereas the dynamic talonavicular joint has a strong stable ligament as well as the medial component of the bifurcate ligament.[30]

Two extrinsic muscle groups provide stability during gait: the peroneal and the posterior tibial muscles. They work synergistically to provide stability. The peroneus brevis and tibialis posterior provide medial/lateral stability and the peroneus longus passes onto the stable cuboid to go from inferior and lateral to a superior and medial attachment to the first ray. This arrangement provides stability of the first ray in propulsion.

The midtarsal joint complex has a pronatory, supinatory axis.[5,24] The oblique axis has a dominant motion in the transverse and sagittal plane and the longitudinal axis has a predominant frontal plane motion. If motion about the oblique axis is not stable, the longitudinal axis allows motion, leading to forefoot supinatus; conversely, if motion around the oblique axis is stable in a supinated position, as in talipes equinovarus, deformity of the longitudinal axis allows forefoot eversion. The latter represents a cavus foot. The former represents a planus foot. Compensatory mechanisms, which occur within the foot secondary to abnormal extrinsic and intrinsic forces, directly influence subtalar and midtarsal function.[5] Abnormal transverse, sagittal, and coronal plane forces must be neutralized for proper foot function from heel strike to toe-off. When conservative management fails to control the foot, surgical intervention is sometimes necessary. Orthotics must be able to control forces in 3 planes. In the frontal plane, posting alone may not be effective when transverse and sagittal plane influences exist. High medial and lateral phalanges extending to the first and fifth metatarsal necks may be necessary. A deep heel seat is also recommended. The University of California Berkeley Laboratories orthosis or the Dynamic Stabilizing Insole System insert control all 3 planes. This advanced insert is both therapeutic and diagnostic. If abnormal forces cannot be controlled or tolerated with orthotics, surgery may have to be considered.

This concept is also important when performing an isolated talonavicular fusion. This fusion is often performed in the adult population for flatfoot reconstruction.[31] When fusing this ball-and-socket joint, it has a dramatic effect on the subtalar joint, limiting its motion by up to 90%.[32] Talonavicular congruity should place the foot slightly pronated to avoid forefoot lateral overload.[33,34] This midtarsal fusion affects the hindfoot as well as the forefoot. Limiting subtalar joint function also affects ankle joint function.[27] In general, fusing major joints has a major impact proximally and distally.

Another major fusion is a triple or double arthrodesis of the rearfoot. It is indicated in more advanced foot deformities and its use alters the architecture of the foot as well as providing stability, which is technically demanding, with special considerations.[35] Adult-acquired flatfoot with associated joint disease, neuromuscular disorders, and posttraumatic conditions are often the indications for these types of fusions. Neuromuscular disorders and posttraumatic conditions as well as congenital anomaly such as clubfoot are also indications for rearfoot fusions.[36–38] Position of fusion is critical, recognizing its influence on the forefoot and ankle. The effect on the ankle is predictable. For example, children born with subtalar, calcaneonavicular, and multiple coalitions may develop ball-and-socket ankle joints because of the loss of torque conversion of the subtalar complex. Functional adaptation of the ankle complex can occur in the younger population, with remodeling of the talus and distal tibiofibular articulations.[16] However, adults develop degenerative joint disease of the ankle because of loss of torque conversion and diminished capability of functional adaptation. Again, a slightly pronated position allows better transition of forces into the forefoot during the propulsive phase of gait. A stable complex after fusion allows better function of the peroneus longus and its effect on the first ray.[13]

The influence of the Achilles tendon and its position when correcting deformity must also be appreciated. This influence is appreciated in Charcot disease, in which the sagittal plane influences the midtarsal and Lisfranc articulations.[39] It must also be considered an adult flatfoot, pediatric flatfoot, and clubfoot deformity. By maintaining proper position with fusions, intrinsic muscles are able to function without positional strain and disease of the peroneal and posterior tibial tendons can be prevented.

In conclusion, various rearfoot fusions, total ankle joint replacements, and normal foot function have been discussed. Experienced biomechanical surgeons must plan carefully, understanding preoperative deformity and intended results. Surgeons try to provide acceptable bipedal locomotion with limited impact as the patient matures. Diagnostic testing, including radiographs, weight-bearing computed tomography scans, and MRI, assists in preoperative planning. Intraoperative fluoroscopy is also essential. Gait analysis is important in evaluating compensatory mechanisms and the position of the foot and leg relative to the progression during gait. Remember that, when building a home, architects and engineers prepare carefully. Lower extremity surgeons are both architects and engineers and apply surgical skills to obtain the most desirable results. An ounce of prevention is worth a pound of cure. The foot is an extremely complex structure that has major effects on the leg, knee, and low back, which also must be taken into consideration when fusion techniques are applied when repositioning of normal function is attempted. Foot and ankle surgeons have the major responsibility of understanding the normal biomechanics of the foot and its influence on the rest of the lower extremity, using the extensive training in the area of biomechanics to apply biomechanical principles to surgical intervention.

REFERENCES

1. Inman VT. The joints of the ankle. Baltimore (MD): Williams & Wilkins; 1976.
2. Zimny S, Schatz H, Pfohl M. The role of limited joint mobility in diabetic patients with an at-risk foot. Diabetes Care 2004;27:942–6.
3. Lavery LA, Armstrong DG, Boulton AJ, et al. Ankle equinus deformity and its relationship to high plantar pressure in a large population with diabetes mellitus. J Am Podiatr Med Assoc 2002;92:479–82.
4. Lowery NJ, Woods JB, Armstrong DG, et al. Surgical management of Charcot neuroarthropathy of the foot and ankle: a systematic review. Foot Ankle Int 2012;33:113–21.
5. Root ML, Orien WP, Weed JH. Normal and abnormal function of the foot. Los Angeles (CA): Clinical Biomechanics Corporation; 1977.
6. Snedeker JG, Wirth SH, Espinosa N. Biomechanics of the normal and arthritic ankle joint. Foot Ankle Clin 2012;17:517–28.
7. Manter JT. Movements of the subtalar and transverse tarsal joints. Anat Rec 1941; 80:397.
8. Mann R, Inman V. Phasic activity of intrinsic muscles of the foot. J Bone Joint Surg Am 1964;46:469–81.
9. Ambagtsheer J. The function of the muscles of the lower leg in relation to movements of the tarsus. Acta Orthop Scand Suppl 1978;172:1–196.
10. Walton L, Villani M. Principles and biomechanical considerations of tendon transfers. Clin Podiatr Med Surg 2016;33(1):1–13.
11. Golanó P, Vega J, de Leeuw PA, et al. Anatomy of the ankle ligaments: a pictorial essay. Knee Surg Sports Traumatol Arthrosc 2010;18:557–69.
12. Saunders JB, Inman V, Eberhart H. The major determinants in normal and pathological gait. J Bone Joint Surg Am 1953;35-A(3):543–58.
13. Johnson C, Christensen J. Biomechanics of the first ray Part 1. The effects of peroneus longus function: a three-dimensional kinematic study on a cadaver model. J Foot Ankle Surg 1999;38(5):313–21.
14. Raikin SM, Sandrowski K, Kane JM, et al. Midterm outcome of the agility total ankle arthroplasty. Foot Ankle Int 2017;38(6):662–70.
15. Gougoulias N, Maffulli N. History of total ankle replacement. Clin Podiatr Med Surg 2013;30:1–20.
16. Bruening D, Cooney TE, Ray MS, et al. Multisegment foot kinematic and kinetic compensations in level and uphill walking following tibiotalar arthrodesis. Foot Ankle Int 2016;37(10):1119–29.
17. Ling JS, Smyth NA, Fraser EJ, et al. Investigating the relationship between ankle arthrodesis and adjacent-joint arthritis in the hindfoot: a systematic review. J Bone Joint Surg Am 2015;97-A(6):513–9.
18. Choi WJ, Yoon HS, Lee JW. Techniques for managing varus and valgus misalignment during total ankle replacement. Clin Podiatr Med Surg 2013;30:35–46.
19. Bartoníček J, Rammelt S, Naňka O. Anatomy of the subtalar joint. Foot Ankle Clin 2018;23(3):315–40.
20. Mittlmeier T, Rammelt S. Update on subtalar joint instability. Foot Ankle Clin 2018; 23(3):397–413.
21. Root ML, Weed JH, Sgarlato TE, et al. Axis of motion of the subtalar joint. An anatomical study. J Am Podiatr Med Assoc 1966;56:149–55.

22. Hill RS. Ankle equinus. Prevalence and linkage to common foot pathology. J Am Podiatr Med Assoc 1995;85:295.

23. Jacobs A, Oloff L. Surgical management of forefoot supinatus in flexible flatfoot deformity. J Foot Surg 1984;23(5):410–49.

24. Elftman H. The transverse tarsal joint and its control. Clin Orthop 1960;16:41–6.

25. Bojsen-Moller F. Calcaneocuboid joint and stability of the longitudinal arch of the foot at high and low gear push off. J Anat 1979;129(1):165–76.

26. Sammarco VJ, Magur EG, Sammarco GJ, et al. Arthrodesis of the subtalar and talonavicular joints for correction of symptomatic hindfoot malalignment. Foot Ankle Int 2006;27:661–6.

27. Catanzariti AR, Mendicino RM, Saltrick KS, et al. Subtalar joint arthrodesis. J Am Podiatr Med Assoc 2005;95:34–41.

28. Weindel S, Schmidt R, Rammelt S, et al. Subtalar instability: a biomechanical cadaver study. Arch Orthop Trauma Surg 2010;130(3):313–9.

29. Jastifer JR, Gustafson PA, Gorman RR. Subtalar arthrodesis alignment: the effect on ankle biomechanics. Foot Ankle Int 2013;34(2):244–50.

30. Walter WR, Hirschmann A, Tafur M, et al. Imaging of chopart (midtarsal) joint complex: normal anatomy and posttraumatic findings. Am J Roentgenol 2018; 211(22):416–25.

31. Fortin P. Posterior tibial tendon insufficiency isolated fusion of the talonavicular joint. Foot Ankle Clin 2001;6:142–4.

32. Astion DJ, Deland JT, Otis JC, et al. Motion of the hindfoot after simulated arthrodesis. J Bone Joint Surg Am 1997;79:241–6.

33. Chen CH, Huang PJ, Chen TB, et al. Isolated talonavicular arthrodesis for talonavicular arthritis. Foot Ankle Int 2001;22:633–6.

34. Fogel GR, Katoh Y, Rand JA, et al. Talonavicular arthrodesis for isolated arthrosis: 9.5 year results and gait analysis. Foot Ankle Int 1982;3:105–13.

35. Angus PD, Cowell HR. Triple arthrodesis. A critical long-term review. J Bone Joint Surg Br 1986;68:260–5.

36. Graves SC, Mann RA, Graves KO. Triple arthrodesis in older adults: results after long-term follow-up. J Bone Joint Surg Am 1993;75:355–62.

37. Saltzman CL, Fehrle MJ, Copper RR, et al. Triple arthrodesis: twenty five and forty four year average follow-up of the same patients. J Bone Joint Surg Am 1999;81: 1391–402.

38. Flemister AS, Infante AF, Sanders RW, et al. Subtalar arthrodesis for complications of intra-articular calcaneal fractures. Foot Ankle Int 2000;21:392–9.

39. Mueller MJ, Sinacore DR, Hastings MK, et al. Effect of Achilles tendon lengthening on neuropathic plantar ulcers. A randomized clinical trial. J Bone Joint Surg Am 2003;85:1436–45.

Pediatric Considerations

Marc A. Benard, DPM[a,b,c,*]

KEYWORDS

- In-toeing • Torsion • Heel-toe • Hyperpronation • Equinus • Reflexes • Infancy
- Galeazzi

KEY POINTS

- The biomechanical assessment of children requires the additional considerations of growth, osseous maturation, gait development, and interpretation of symptoms conveyed by the child.
- Performing and interpreting the biomechanical examination in children depends on an understanding of both the cognitive ability of the child and clinical norms and normal variations achieved at particular ages.
- Radiographic assessment in young children is limited by incomplete ossification or lack of ossification and the clinician must rely more on the physical examination and history presented.
- The plasticity of tissue with growth and development in children is an advantage when observation or conservative treatment is rendered; however, this also requires more frequent interval assessment in children than in adults.

OVERVIEW

The focus of this article is on understanding the nuances that the practitioner must be aware of to effectively assess and/or treat children biomechanically, be the intervention surgical, nonsurgical, or a combination. The intent is to raise practitioner awareness of this subset of patients and, where helpful, to provide clinical pearls and insights to aid in patient management. The focus is not to provide lists of pediatric or radiographic norms or therapeutic modalities, because these can easily be ascertained elsewhere.

INTRODUCTION

In this special article, *Clinics In Podiatric Medicine and Surgery* invited Marc A. Benard, DPM, to answer a short series of questions about the important considerations when taking care of pediatric patients with lower extremity complaints. For many providers,

Disclosure Statement: The author has nothing to disclose.
[a] Baja Project for Crippled Children/Operation Footprint, Westlake Village, CA, USA; [b] American Board of Podiatric Medicine, Hermosa Beach, CA, USA; [c] Western University of Podiatric Medicine, Pomona, CA, USA
* 1352 Richmond Road, Jackson Springs, NC 27281.
E-mail address: mbenard@abpmed.org

the biomechanical evaluation of children is very difficult because younger patients are different from adults and have very different needs and require a different approach by providers. As such, Dr Benard is an excellent resource for physicians with this complex class of patients. Dr Benard is Co-director of the Baja Project For Crippled Children/Operation Footprint, which has been rendering humanitarian foot and ankle care to children in Mexico, El Salvador, and Honduras since 1976 and has trained hundreds of podiatric residents from programs throughout the nation. With more than 37 years of practice and lecture experience, he is recognized nationally as an educator in clinical biomechanics with an emphasis on the nonsurgical and surgical treatment of children with lower extremity disorders.

WHAT IMPORTANT GENERAL FACTORS ARE UNIQUE TO CHILDREN WITH LOWER EXTREMITY COMPLAINTS?

Although the application of biomechanical principles in children, both for surgical and nonsurgical intervention, is equally necessary as that for adults, significant differences exist with respect to:

- Growth
- Osseous maturation
- Gait development
- Interpretation of symptoms conveyed by the child

Growth

The plasticity of growing tissue offers the practitioner the advantage of a more responsive tissue adaptation to the alteration of forces produced by the given intervention, be it serial casting, bracing (orthoses) or surgery. Appropriately used, this advantage must include the practitioner's knowledge of pediatric norms of development.

- What is the normal range and gender variation of joint motion and position for a given age group?
- What are the age-adjusted pediatric norms for hip, femur, knee, tibia, tarsal, lesser tarsal, and metatarsal positions?
- When can the child be expected to move to an "improved" position regardless of (ie, despite) outside intervention?
- When is watchful waiting sufficient, and when is the appropriate time to intervene based on windows of opportunity either afforded by growth or as a result of its cessation?
- To what extent does body mass and the amount of residual or acquired body fat have on the type of foot or ankle–foot device chosen?

Yet another level of practitioner awareness must be applied when faced with neurologically impacted children, where the neurologic condition may affect normal joint position and motion, or responsiveness to treatment.

Osseous Maturation

Osseous maturation factor applies to both diagnostic as well as therapeutic modalities.

Imaging

As a result of areas of radiographic silence in the foot and ankle for younger children (prewalkers, toddlers, early walkers and even heel-toe walkers) the practitioner must, in many cases, rely on the relative positioning of partially ossified bone to assess the pre-, intra-, and postintervention effectiveness. In **Fig. 1**, for example, the navicular, along with most of the lesser tarsus, is not visualized in this infant with metatarsus adductus. The biomechanical assessment is therefore primarily clinical; however, based on the degree of rigidity, clinical course, concurrent musculoskeletal findings elsewhere, and responsiveness to care, imaging studies can assist the practitioner in decision making.

For example, a child undergoing manipulation and serial casting for recalcitrant metatarsus adductus should be periodically assessed radiologically during the course of treatment to make sure that the reduction is occurring properly at the midfoot (relationship between the first or second ray bisection to the calcaneal bisection) rather than a spurious correction, where the reduction is occurring more proximally, via cuboid abduction on the calcaneus or an increase in Kite's angle. Clinically, the foot may appear the same whether the reduction is correct or incorrect.

Similarly, other conditions in children are best assessed biomechanically with a combination of clinical and radiographic parameters. In **Fig. 2** a child with a beginning toe–heel gait pattern shows plantarflexion with some flattening of the trochlear surface of the talus. Often the flattening is not evident, as the talus is not completely ossified. Therefore, the practitioner must rely on nonradiographic parameters to determine if the ankle joint limitation is due to other factors (eg, tight posterior ankle joint capsule and ligaments, etc).

Although radiographs can be valuable in primary evaluation and for periodic monitoring of a child over time, and as osseous maturity makes structures more visible, the clinical biomechanical evaluation of the child is essential.

WHAT CONSIDERATIONS ARE IMPORTANT WHEN EVALUATING CHILDREN'S GAIT PATTERNS?

Gait assessment in children requires additional interpretive skills owing to functional and structural changes concurrent with their normal growth and neurologic

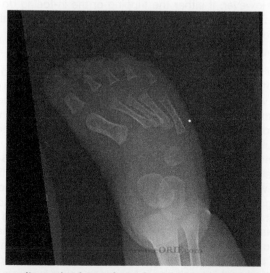

Fig. 1. Dorsoplantar radiograph of an infant's foot demonstrating physiologic absence of most of the lesser tarsus. (*From* M. Benard, DPM. Differential Diagnosis of Metatarsus Adductus. Podiatry Management 2014;33:139-44; with permission.)

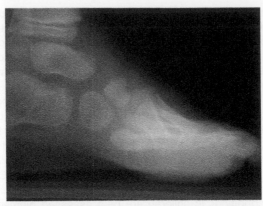

Fig. 2. Plantarflexed foot position with adaptative flattening of talar trochlear surface.

maturation. Essentially, the practitioner must know what is developmentally normal, or within normal variation at a particular age, to assess what is abnormal. Broadly, the initial questions to be asked are as follows.

- When did the child begin weight bearing or ambulating?
  - If delayed, is this an isolated finding or does a pattern of developmental delay exist (ie, at what age did independent head control, sitting, standing, verbalization, etc, occur)?
- If the onset of ambulation is temporally within normal limits, is the child's gait pattern toe to toe, toe to heel, foot-flat to foot-flat, or heel to toe? Is the demonstrated gait pattern age appropriate?
  - For example, toe walking in children is common and self-corrects with age. However, its persistence beyond age 3 demands a neurologic assessment.
  - Tripping or falling, common in children who are in-toed, normally self-corrects with age. However, if either the tripping or the in-toeing do not self-correct, or if the in-toeing corrects via hyperpronation (ie, compensation) and the original source remains, then further workup or therapeutic intervention are warranted.

The presence or absence of an active gait and the type of gait can often dictate the nature of therapeutic intervention. Nonambulatory children are often good candidates for serial casting when intervention is necessary. In contrast, shoes and orthoses, where indicated, are, in most cases, better suited when the child encounters ground reactive force, and more so when the gait cycle attains definitive heel contact, midstance, and propulsive phases.

For example, recalcitrant internal tibial torsion or position in a 6-month-old baby could respond well to a course of serial casting, whereas a child first presenting at 15 months of age would have a much more challenging, if any, response to that intervention. Assuming intervention is warranted, the latter child would not yet have adopted a heel-toe gait pattern and would therefore not require a level of customization of foot orthoses if this modality were chosen. In this example, if orthoses are chosen, or some other form of dynamic bracing, is the intent to alter the actual angle of gait, to stabilize the child against tripping and falling, or both? If the child presents at age 7 with a fully developed heel-toe gait and is becoming active in sports, is the goal treatment of secondary compensation (eg, at the foot, knee or hip level), referral for assessment by another specialist, or both?

In summary, the same condition in separate age brackets, with different capacities for ambulation and levels of activity, may be treated differently. In addition, from a treatment perspective, in ambulatory children it is the combination of orthotic type and shoes that define the environment in which the foot is placed that should be considered.

Children of an appropriate cognitive level will often attempt to walk correctly when prompted to walk by the practitioner. Sometimes they are even encouraged by their parents or caregivers to do so. The practitioner should anticipate this and either find a good way to distract the child while they walk to eliminate their posturing or wait until the child's gait is free of behavioral posturing before its assessment is undertaken.

WHAT PRACTITIONER SKILLS ARE HELPFUL WHEN INTERPRETING SYMPTOMS CONVEYED BY THE CHILD?

In the larger context, evaluating and treating children requires another layer of skills beyond the clinical. Three skills in particular are needed:

- The ability to tailor history taking and physical assessment to the cognitive and communicative capability of children of different ages. The practitioner must often elicit information in another way from children because of these differences. Much of the physical examination, biomechanical or otherwise, requires communication for the requested response, or motion, in a way that the child of a given age can understand and/or with which they have the capacity to comply. For example, an infant still exhibiting the special reflexes of infancy may be adequately muscle tested by assessing an assortment of them. A 3-year-old child may be muscle tested by using certain phrases such as, for example, "can you walk like a duck?" or asking them to duplicate a motion that the provider demonstrates.
- The ability to interpret children's responses appropriately and understand that the descriptors of clinical symptoms are often different for children than adults. Children may not describe discomfort (or pain) similarly to adults; instead they may modify their behavior. A simple but common example would be a young child asking to be carried because they are tired. Older children may avoid physical activity, but are nonspecific as to why.
- The ability to assess physical findings quickly and at times unconventionally based on the limited attention span and cooperation of the child. This may require altering the position of the child for making the assessment, or engaging the parent during the examination or treatment process. The younger the child, the more this strategy becomes necessary.

WHAT ARE THE IMPORTANT METHODS AND CONSIDERATIONS WHEN PERFORMING A BIOMECHANICAL EXAMINATION ON A CHILD?

In children, a biomechanical examination and a general musculoskeletal, or neuromuscular examination, are essentially synonymous, especially with infants, prewalkers, and early walkers. Once a heel-to-toe gait is assumed, the generally accepted biomechanical examination undertakes the elements generally used in the adult population, with these caveats:

- The interpretation of findings must be made in the context of angulatory changes occurring with normal growth and development.
- The effective assessment of the child biomechanically rests largely on the ability to gain or elicit the cooperation of the child. This could require that the child is

examined at a time when the child is most cooperative. In essence, behavioral observation or modification may be required to perform the examination effectively.

As an overview, it is useful to divide the examination into prewalkers (neonates and infants), foot-flat to foot-flat walkers (toddlers and early walkers), and heel-toe walkers.

Prewalkers

Neonates and infants should be assessed grossly for symmetry of motion in joint range and quality, as well as in resting position. The spine should be assessed and palpated for a rectus position. In normal infants and newborns the spine is central without curvature in the frontal or transverse planes, and the gluteal folds are symmetric. Gluteal folds are a convenient external marker because, when they seems to be asymmetric, further clinical assessment of the hip is needed.

Hip assessment

Ortolani's, Barlow's, and telescoping (Galeazzi) examinations are normally used. The resting position of the hip in newborns and infants is mildly flexed and abducted, but there should be no restriction of adduction and internal rotation when the hip is placed through its range of motion. The hip is taken through flexion, abduction/adduction, and internal/external rotation. Because the flexed, abducted, externally rotated hip is in its most stable position, if the hip can be dislocated from this position (Barlow's test), further intervention (pillowing, abduction splintage, etc) may be required. Clicking felt in the hip joint when moving the femur into abduction from a flexed position may be indicative of a dislocated femoral head that is being relocated into the acetabulum (Ortolani's sign). Telescoping, or posterior dislocation with the hip in an innately less stable position (flexed and adducted), is indicative of the femoral head moving out of the acetabulum with anterior pressure and then relocating when relaxed or drawn forward.

Abduction of the hip position reduces with age. Human infants are adapted with an abducted position to create a broadened base for stability on weight bearing.

Knee assessment

The knee should be assessed in all 3 planes. Bilateral symmetry is expected; however, in prewalkers (newborns and infants) the retention of intrauterine position results in mild knee flexion at rest, which should be easily reducible on examination to a rectus position. This gradually reduces with age. The knee should be stable in the frontal plane and in a rectus attitude; however, this position is often misinterpreted by the practitioner owing to the natural combination of external hip position, knee flexion and mild internal tibial torsion, or position, which makes the knee seem to be in varus.

Tibial torsion or position is clinically internal relative to the femur, and its internal position gradually reduces with age. Although tibial torsion is an osseous finding and tibial position is not, in young children and prewalkers they usually occur concurrently and are managed in the same way. Positional conditions can be acquired from sleeping and sitting habits. In prewalkers, assessment of the transverse plane is important, although its clinical significance is more relevant when the child becomes ambulatory, because children in older age groups are often presented with issues of tripping. This topic is discussed with the older age bracket.

Ankle range of motion in newborns and infants is significantly greater than adults, especially in dorsiflexion. The dorsum of the foot in normal infants can be made to touch the tibia with gentle pressure. Older literature can be misleading in correlating this finding with talipes calcaneovalgus (**Fig. 3**) or congenital vertical talus (**Figs. 4 and 5**); however, from the clinician's perspective the degree of normal dorsiflexion

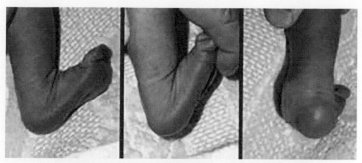

Fig. 3. Clinical appearance of talipes calcaneovalgus.

is more a matter of the amount of effort required to dorsiflex the foot to the tibia. Resting position of the ankle in newborns and infants should be neutral to mild plantarflexion. Of significance, however, is where the resting position is dorsiflexed, and the dorsum of the foot can be quite easily brought to the tibia. In that case, talipes calcaneovalgus or vertical talus should be ruled out.

Talipes calcaneovalgus usually reduces spontaneously and treatment is rarely needed. Recalcitrant cases may undergo a short course of serial casting. Of greater concern in this age bracket is a limitation of ankle dorsiflexion. When neonates or infants can be brought only to perpendicular, or less, the source of the equinus must be determined, because it is never normal. Typically, 45° or more of ankle dorsiflexion is expected. Therefore, when a neonate or infant shows ankle dorsiflexion even in the normal adult range, the condition should be pursued further (see **Figs. 3–5**).

Subtalar range of motion in prewalkers should be assessed grossly for symmetry and smooth range. Neonates have little adipose tissue to obscure the bony contours, and limitation of subtalar motion is easily detected. Note that residual intrauterine position may maintain the foot in mild supination at rest, but the position should easily reduce on examination to a neutral or pronated position, with the heel everting relative to the distal leg. Note, however, that as the child begins to acquire baby fat the contours around the foot and ankle are less distinct in the frontal plane, and subtalar resting position and range of motion are better obtained by palpating the heel medially and laterally and feeling for the calcaneal position rather than relying on visual assessment.

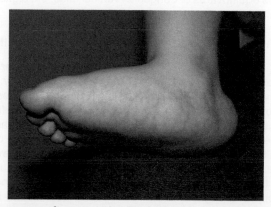

Fig. 4. Clinical appearance of congenital vertical talus.

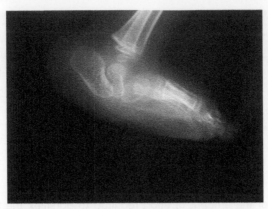

Fig. 5. Lateral non-weight bearing image of congenital vertical talus.

In prewalkers, a triplanar assessment of the midfoot should be performed; however, particular attention should be paid to the transverse and frontal planes, because a globally plantarflexed (or dorsiflexed) forefoot, or plantarflexed first ray, is not normally encountered. When a sagittal midfoot abnormality is noted in this age bracket, it rarely occurs in isolation and is typically associated with hindfoot and ankle pathology, such as with a congenital or neurologic condition, for example, talipes equinovarus, congenital vertical talus, or possibly oblique talus.

Absent pathology of that nature, transverse plane assessment of the forefoot should easily demonstrate abduction beyond a rectus lateral border. Metatarsus adductus is a common condition wherein the lateral border may not be easily brought to rectus, or brought to rectus with significant resistance. Typically, this transverse plane condition resolves spontaneously with weight bearing, or via gentle manipulation, if recalcitrant. Be advised that if intervention through manipulation is undertaken with splintage (cast or taping), it is important to avoid pronating, rather than just abducting, the forefoot on the hindfoot, which can compromise the stability of the lateral column.

In prewalkers, digits are assessed grossly, because developmental digital contracture is rare. When contracture is encountered, it typically presents congenitally (eg, curly toe, digital elevatus of the second toe). Even in conditions of a more global nature, such as talipes equinovarus or congenital vertical talus, the digits are typically in a rectus attitude.

IS THERE A PRACTICAL WAY TO ASSESS MUSCLE STRENGTH IN AN INFANT?

Muscle testing in prewalkers, especially in neonates and younger infants, can be accomplished through assessment of the special reflexes of infancy. The practitioner should be familiar with and able to perform them. The special reflexes of infancy are a suite of pattern movements elicited by specific stimuli and are a useful way to grossly assess symmetry and range of motion, while in part also evaluating the child neurologically. Although the full expression of a specific reflex is not always obtained, or may have disappeared based on the age of the child, judicious use of several of these reflexes can provide an excellent assessment of the child's biomechanical and neuromuscular status. In addition, persistence of these reflexes at an age when they should have disappeared may be indicative of developmental delay and may be clinically significant in patient management. Therefore, their assessment is important beyond the sole purpose of biomechanical evaluation. Some of the most useful are as follows.

- *Babinski*—The sole of the infant or child's foot is stroked, causing the hallux to dorsiflex and the lesser toes to fan. When fully expressed (not always demonstrated) the ankle will dorsiflex and the knee will flex. This reflex extinguishes by approximately age 2.
- *Walking or step reflex*—The infant is held upright and when the foot touches a solid surface the extremity withdraws and then extends back to the surface. This reflex helps to evaluate multiple muscle groups simultaneously and is useful for assessment of sagittal motion at the hip, knee and ankle. This reflex typically extinguishes by age 4 to 6 months.
- *Moro or startle reflex*—The reflex is elicited by startling the infant by a loud sound, resulting in backward neck extension, abduction of the arms, and extension of the legs, followed by flexion of the arms and legs. When fully elicited, many muscle groups and joints can be assessed simultaneously. The reflex extinguishes at about age 5 to 6 months.
- *Tonic neck reflex*—The infant's head is turned to one side and the arm on that side extends, while the contralateral arm flexes at the elbow. This reflex extinguishes at about 6 to 7 months of age.
- *Righting reflex*—With the infant supine, the head is brought to one side and the shoulders and trunk respond by rotating to the same side. This reflex extinguishes by age 1 year.
- *Grasping reflex*—The infant's palm is stroked and the fingers reflexively flex. This reflex extinguishes at about age 5 to 6 months.

When muscle testing children who have matured beyond the special reflexes of infancy, the challenge is obtaining the needed information when the child is unwilling or cognitively incapable to follow a directive. At this time, observation of the child's movements, via play with a toy or other object of interest (eg, neuro hammer, touch screen, etc), or through their frank muscle resistance to the practitioner's hands-on assessment can accomplish the task of muscle testing effectively. In essence, the practitioner is examining the area of interest indirectly, or at least unconventionally.

Biomechanical Assessment at Ages 1 Through 3 or 4 Years

This covers the time when the child normally is weight bearing and becoming more active in gait. It is a rather broad time frame, when growth is rapid and, as indicated, requires an understanding of musculoskeletal developmental norms. The practitioner must have an appropriate frame of reference for a given age so that prudent decision making, that is, watchful waiting versus intervention, can be made.

Within this age range and beyond, children differ in the natural reduction of, or change in, foot and lower extremity angles, as well as flexibility. In addition, the epidemic of childhood obesity in the United States or other nations adopting the so-called Western diet has introduced another variable leading to increased pes planus and more proximal issues, such as increased physiologic bowing of the tibia.

Transverse plane conditions leading to parental concern (eg, tripping and falling, cosmetic, etc) are often encountered by the practitioner. The natural reduction of external femoral position and internal tibial torsion in children do not necessarily occur concurrently with precision and residual in-toeing is common. Therefore, segmental assessment is required to determine the source (or sources) of the adduction, which may be osseous, soft tissue, or both. This assessment is needed to guide patient care and to communicate with the parents. Patients with a neurologic history introduce yet another variable, because often the static, or open chain assessment may differ from the gait findings, where upper motor neuron influences may manifest that have not been detected with manual muscle testing or range of motion assessment.

Torsional or rotational conditions are often best assessed by first observing the child's gait, where symmetry with respect to angle of gait, cadence, and stride length are easily assessed. Where concurrent frontal plane deviations are present (eg, genuvarum or genuvalgum) the base of the gait is better appreciated dynamically than with the child in static stance. During gait, the patellae are convenient landmarks for determining whether the source of in-toeing is emanating from the femur or hip joint. In most cases, if the patellae are observed to be oscillating close to the sagittal plane the source of the in-toeing is distal (ie, in the tibia, midfoot, or both). Corroboration should be made via non-weight bearing assessment, where segmental evaluation (hip range of motion, both flexed and extended, transverse motion at the knee, assessment of the thigh–foot axis, assessment of the midfoot) will help to determine the location(s) contributing to the in-toeing. In children who have developed a heel-to-toe gait pattern, if the in-toeing is asymmetric during gait then assessment of limb length should be made as the potential source of the asymmetry. In addition, in heel-to-toe walkers who are in-toed, assess for hamstring tightness. Although gastrocnemius or gastrocsoleus tightness is rare in children (other than those with neurologic conditions) medial hamstring tightness is common and sometimes contributory to the adducted angle of gait. Therefore, do not neglect this assessment and, if the condition is present, consider a stretching program, if practical, in the management plan.

Early walkers or foot-flat to foot-flat walkers who are in-toed infrequently exhibit posterior hamstring tightness. The most common source of their in-toeing is at the tibia. This will be determined with segmental evaluation, previously described elsewhere in this article. As discussed elsewhere in this article, a common error in assessment, however, is mistaking internal tibial torsion for genu varum (**Fig. 6**). This misinterpretation happens because the presence of baby fat (or exogenous obesity in older children) creates an optical illusion wherein the outer calf is more visible than the inner calf when viewing the patient from anterior. This can create the appearance of varum at or near the knee, where none exists. Another common error is to mistake this for tibial varum when none is present. The significance of a misdiagnosis is that, although internal tibial torsion is typically a benign condition usually outgrown, genu varum (idiopathic tibia vara) requires a higher level of scrutiny and possible intervention. Note that the latter differs from physiologic bowing of the tibia, which is typically present and likewise outgrown. Also note that although internal tibial torsion is usually outgrown, heel-toe walkers often compensate for the resulting in-toeing through excessive foot pronation. This compensation can mask the problem or lead the practitioner to a misdiagnosis or incomplete diagnosis of the condition. If treatment is undertaken, it should be directed to eliminating the compensation until the tibial segment corrects.

Clinical Pearls

Pragmatically, and for ease of assessment, consider initiating the examination with gait analysis if the child is ambulatory and cooperative. Much of the information needed is gained during gait observation, with corroboration of non-weight bearing and stance findings and, if the child is in shoes, their evaluation. In addition, placing the child prone during the non-weight bearing examination has the advantage of their facing their parent or caregiver at the head of the table and not looking at the provider, which

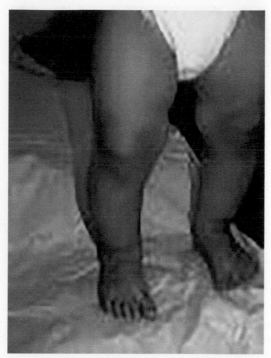

Fig. 6. Clinical appearance of internal tibial torsion. Note the intoed appearance despite an externally rotated thigh. (*From* M. Benard, DPM. Differential Diagnosis of Metatarsus Adductus. Podiatry Management 2014;33:139-44; with permission.)

both eases them and eliminates their anticipation of the practitioner moving their lower extremities and feet in a particular direction. Furthermore, much of the needed information can be obtained in that position, including hip assessment in the transverse and sagittal plane, as well as segmental assessment of the femur, tibia, ankle, hindfoot, and midfoot. In the prone position the hips are automatically extended and, when the knees are flexed at 90°, it is easy to imagine the lower legs (tibia) as arms on a clock face. Because each number on a clock face is 30° from the next, this strategy facilitates visualization, and differences of 5° or even less can be seen without the use of external measuring devices. Counterrotating the left and right extremities internally and externally and "reading the time" allows for easy assessment of asymmetry in femoral rotation both between the 2 limbs and within each limb as well.

Femoral anteversion (**Fig. 7**) is the most common cause of in-toeing in early childhood. Femoral anteversion is defined by the relation between the femoral neck and the transcondylar axis at the knee. It is normal at birth and reduces with age, but, if delayed, may be a cause of tripping or awkward gait in children and is commonly the reason for parental presentation of the child. The condition's normal course results in near complete resolution by adolescence.

The functional significance for the practitioner is in making a thorough segmental assessment. A simple clinical assessment method in ambulatory children is to observe the patellae as the child approaches during gait. The patellae will be internal to the sagittal plane. Femoral anteversion may be the source, or a contributory element, of the child's adducted angle of gait. The clinician should be aware that children commonly pronate in compensation for the adduction, which may mask another condition such as persistent metatarsus adductus. A comparison should therefore be

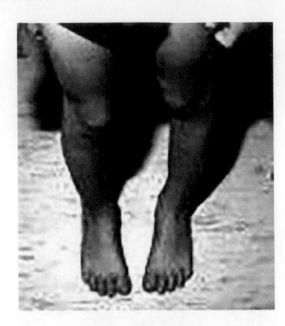

Fig. 7. Clinical appearance of femoral anteversion. (*From* M. Benard, DPM. Differential Diagnosis of Metatarsus Adductus. Podiatry Management 2014;33:139-44; with permission.)

made with the feet in their compensated stance position and corrected stance position (with both feet placed in neutral stance). If metatarsus adductus (or forefoot adductus) is present, it will become more evident.

Tibial torsion or position can be assessed in the same prone, knee-flexed position while keeping the ankle and foot neutral (**Fig. 8**, thigh–foot angle). This position eliminates the influence of the hip, femur, and, absent abnormal midfoot adduction, the foot. It helps to isolate the transverse position of the lower leg for assessment.

Internal tibial torsion is a normal condition in infants and is present through 18 to 24 months of age. It is defined by the relationship of the leg to the thigh and typically resolves spontaneously. Where the thigh–foot angle is internal and exceeds –10° at 24 months, monitoring, though not necessarily treatment, is warranted. Intervention, where indicated, is most often accomplished through dynamic bracing (eg, Wheaton type, or analogous bracing, which maintains an abductory force on the tibia with the knee in a flexed position). Clinicians advocating intervention do so on the basis of decreased tripping and falling in ambulatory children. Older therapies, such as abductory bars at the foot level only, are less effective and tend to shift the moment of force to the femur rather than where it is intended.

A convenient clinical assessment of internal tibial position can be made with the child facing the examiner as the leg is internally and externally rotated relative to the thigh with the knee flexed at 90° and the foot held in neutral. An internal tibial position, or torsion, results in the foot being more adducted than abducted relative to the patella when the leg is taken through a range of motion.

Assessment of Foot Adduction

The persistence of metatarsus adductus can play a role in the overall in-toeing of the child, both as an isolated entity or in combination of other areas contributing to the in-toeing. The foot is C shaped with a convex lateral border and concave medial border (**Fig. 9**).

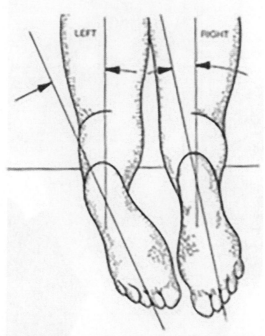

Fig. 8. Measurement representation of the thigh–foot angle. (*From* M. Benard, DPM. Differential Diagnosis of Metatarsus Adductus. Podiatry Management 2014;33:139-44; with permission.)

Although the vast majority of cases are flexible and typically resolve spontaneously a spectrum of flexibility exists, from semirigid to rigid. In the context of in-toeing, for that reason, the condition bears attention with respect to its diagnosis and management. Most children require only periodic monitoring of the condition, without additional foot radiographs. In addition, a small percentage of cases are associated with hip dysplasia and evaluation of hip stability should be part of the biomechanical assessment. Much of the radiographic information otherwise available in adults is silent or only partially available in children (see **Fig. 1**). From a biomechanical perspective, therefore, metatarsus adductus is clinically indistinguishable from forefoot adductus in prewalkers and beyond, and they are evaluated and managed in the same way.

Practically speaking, the preponderance of children presenting for the condition are prewalkers and the biomechanical assessment entails abduction of the forefoot on the hindfoot, evaluating the ease of manual reduction. Flexible presentations are typified by the forefoot being easily manipulated into a rectus or mildly abducted position (**Figs. 10** and **11**).

Care should be taken to abduct rather than pronate the forefoot, because iatrogenic forefoot pronation will lead the practitioner into a false sense of its reducibility. In semirigid or rigid conditions, or conditions recalcitrant to care, the practitioner should evaluate cutaneous landmarks, such as creases in the mid-arch and posterior ankle, because these entities are common with talipes equinovarus (**Figs. 12–14**). From a biomechanical perspective the differentiation of the 2 conditions is essential, because the latter is a more significant condition and requires treatment and close monitoring.

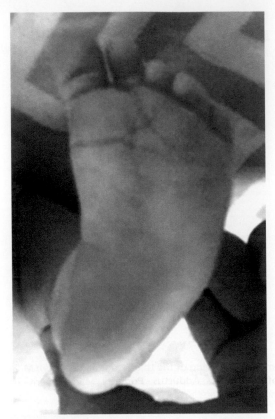

Fig. 9. Clinical appearance of metatarsus adductus with concave medial and convex lateral foot borders. (*From* M. Benard, DPM. Differential Diagnosis of Metatarsus Adductus. Podiatry Management 2014;33:139-44; with permission.)

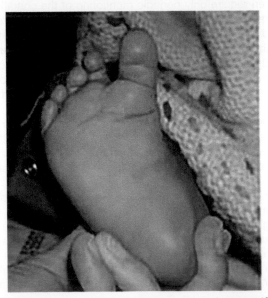

Fig. 10. Examination of metatarsus adductus. (*From* M. Benard, DPM. Differential Diagnosis of Metatarsus Adductus. Podiatry Management 2014;33:139-44; with permission.)

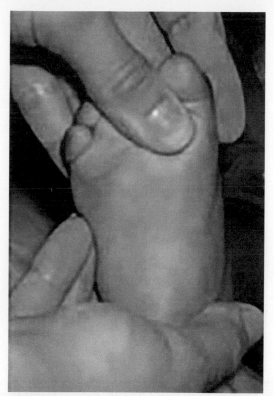

Fig. 11. Reduction of deformity indicating flexible metatarsus adductus. (*From* M. Benard, DPM. Differential Diagnosis of Metatarsus Adductus. Podiatry Management 2014;33:139-44; with permission.)

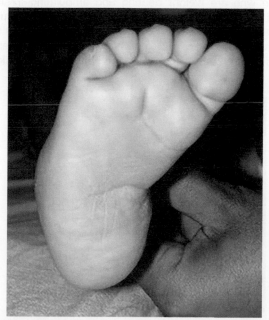

Fig. 12. Clinical appearance of the multiplanar nature of talipes equinovarus. (*From* M. Benard, DPM. Differential Diagnosis of Metatarsus Adductus. Podiatry Management 2014;33:139–44; with permission.)

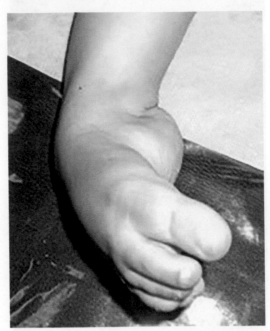

Fig. 13. Clinical appearance of the multiplanar nature of talipes equinovarus. (*From* M. Benard, DPM. Differential Diagnosis of Metatarsus Adductus. Podiatry Management 2014;33:139-44; with permission.)

In older children who are weight bearing and ambulating, residual metatarsus adductus can lead to pronatory compensation at the hindfoot and mild forefoot supinatus, mandating appropriate radiographs to assess Kite's ankle as well as the talar–first metatarsal relationship. These radiographs are important in differentiating persistent metatarsus adductus (compensated or uncompensated) from skewfoot, in which

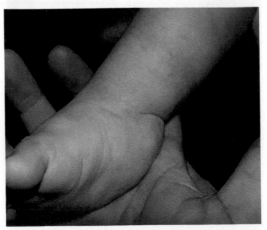

Fig. 14. Clinical appearance of the multiplanar nature of talipes equinovarus. (*From* M. Benard, DPM. Differential Diagnosis of Metatarsus Adductus. Podiatry Management 2014;33:139-44; with permission.)

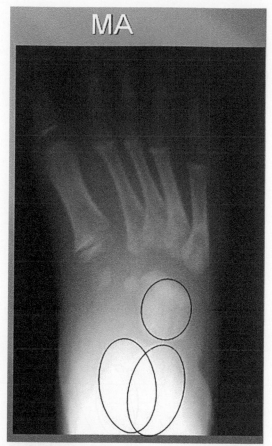

Fig. 15. Dorsoplantar radiographs of metatarsus adductus, talipes equinovarus, and skew-foot. (*From* M. Benard, DPM. Differential Diagnosis of Metatarsus Adductus. Podiatry Management 2014;33:139-44; with permission.)

the tarsals are excessively pronated, or talipes equinovarus, in which the tarsals are excessively supinated (**Fig. 15**, a dorsoplantar radiograph of metatarsus adductus; **Fig. 16**, a dorsoplantar radiograph of talipes equinovarus; and **Fig. 17**, a dorsoplantar radiograph of skewfoot).

The hallux is often adducted as well and can be exaggerated with weight bearing (**Fig. 18**).

The scope of this article precludes a detailed review of talipes equinovarus and skewfoot, both complex deformities, and the reader is encouraged to familiarize themselves with them. As discussed elsewhere in this article, the presence of adipose tissue can mask in children what would otherwise be readily observable in teenagers or adults. Of particular importance is the need for the clinician to perform a thorough biomechanical assessment, with radiographs as needed, to be able to differentiate among the 3 conditions and make appropriate management decisions. As a practical example, undetected hindfoot supination causes resistance to manual abduction of the forefoot, leading to a misunderstanding of the etiology of its motion and (adducted) position. Undetected hindfoot pronation can lead to the reverse, that is, an impression

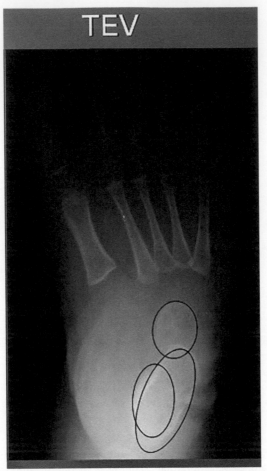

Fig. 16. Dorsoplantar radiographs of metatarsus adductus, talipes equinovarus, and skew-foot. (*From* M. Benard, DPM. Differential Diagnosis of Metatarsus Adductus. Podiatry Management 2014;33:139-44; with permission.)

of hypermobility of the forefoot and midfoot as a cause of the pronatory condition rather than the hindfoot.

Assessment of Ankle Joint Dorsiflexion

In children from about age 3 years on, ankle joint dorsiflexion is more easily assessed with the child prone. Before that age, they are typically being held or sitting with their parents or care givers during the examination. Although assessment in adults can also be performed prone, in children this helps to eliminate anticipation by the child when approached by the examiner, which often influences the tone of the posterior muscles. From the prone, knee-flexed position (**Fig. 19**), the gastrocnemius and hamstrings are not stretched when the ankle is dorsiflexed, and ankle dorsiflexion is much less subject to their influence. Beginning from the knee flexed position the child will not then anticipate when the knee is extended (**Fig. 20**). This method provides a more reliable assessment in pediatric patients

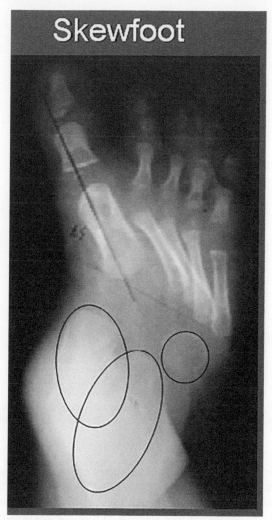

Fig. 17. Dorsoplantar radiographs of metatarsus adductus, talipes equinovarus, and skew-foot. (*From* M. Benard, DPM. Differential Diagnosis of Metatarsus Adductus. Podiatry Management 2014;33:139-44; with permission.)

and eliminates false-positive diagnoses of gastrocnemius equinus. Absent abnormal upper motor neuron influence, if ankle dorsiflexion is deficient via this method, the deficiency is likely present.

Hindfoot Assessment

The adipose tissue in the lower leg and heel area of young children who are weight bearing or ambulatory renders the precise stance or gait evaluation of hindfoot position difficult. Nor is that level of precision required. When visible, however, the Achilles tendon can be a useful indirect marker for subtalar position. Its central position relative to the posterior ankle or lower leg is consistent with a neutral hindfoot position. If the tendon seems to be medial to the midline, the hindfoot is pronated and if lateral to the midline the foot is supinated.

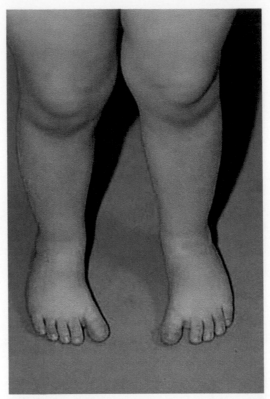

Fig. 18. Clinical weightbearing appearance of hallux adductus/hallux varus. (*From* M. Benard, DPM. Differential Diagnosis of Metatarsus Adductus. Podiatry Management 2014;33:139-44; with permission.)

A common error made in the stance assessment of rearfoot position, regardless of the child's age, is the practitioner's failure to adjust their viewing position properly relative to the posterior leg and heel. Habitually, gait or stance is assessed from directly anterior and posterior. Although this vantage is important, concurrent assessment of each limb individually helps to detect asymmetry. As shown in **Fig. 21**, bilateral hindfoot position is viewed from directly posterior. The left hindfoot seems to be slightly more pronated than the right. If, however, each hindfoot is viewed individually and from the proper angle, as shown in **Figs. 22** and **23**, the amount of asymmetry is readily appreciated. This finding is important relative to both diagnosis and treatment and can mean the difference between monitoring a condition or initiating treatment.

Midfoot Assessment

In both ambulatory children and adults, instability at the midfoot is subject to planal dominance. When midfoot motion is primarily transverse plane dominated, the resulting "too many toes" sign is present, which is commonly described as the forefoot being abducted on the hindfoot. In reality, because both the forefoot and hindfoot are maintained on the ground by frictional forces, transverse plane midfoot motion is due to adduction of the talus as it is rotated medially with the ankle mortise along with the leg's rotation. This finding is clinically significant, because this foot type usually demonstrates little excess frontal plane motion at the hindfoot. Unlike frontal plane

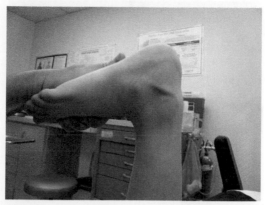

Fig. 19. Ankle dorsiflexion with knee flexed.

deviations at the midfoot or forefoot, which can adapt with age and angulatory changes elsewhere, this condition does not change with age. Where indicated, treatment via orthoses, surgery, or both needs to be directed at midfoot control. Controlling the hindfoot alone can still result in midfoot instability in midstance and propulsion.

When midfoot motion is primarily frontal plane dominated and the forefoot is found to be in varus or supinatus relative to the hindfoot, which is common in children, compensation is usually noted at the subtalar joint via hyperpronation. As noted elsewhere in this article, this condition can often be asymptomatic and self-correcting over time. Where intervention is warranted, alignment of the hindfoot to leg relationship with orthoses or, if severe enough, surgery, should be aimed at reducing hindfoot pronation, which narrows Kite's angle and realigns the talonavicular joint. At that point, the plasticity innate to the child's growth will result in midfoot realignment.

Sagittal plane dominance at the midfoot in children is often due to neurologic influence, for example, with cerebral palsy, causing hypertonicity, a supinated hindfoot, a narrowed Kite's angle, increased transverse tarsal arch and medial longitudinal arch and equinus that can be functional, soft tissue, or both. This foot type is typically cavo-adducto-varus. Typically, the first ray is plantarflexed, resulting in a valgus forefoot to rearfoot relationship, which can be exacerbated over time if lateral column overload leads to dorsal

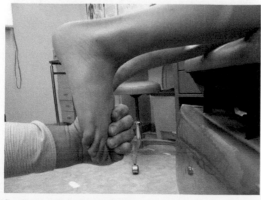

Fig. 20. Ankle dorsiflexion with knee extended.

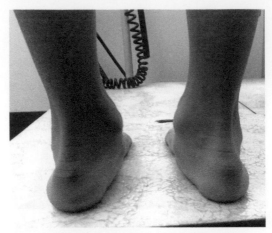

Fig. 21. Bilateral hindfoot appearance from directly posterior.

subluxation of the fifth metatarsal or, on occasion, the fourth and fifth metatarsals. The clinician is advised to pay close attention to developing cavo-adducto-varus feet in young children who otherwise seem to be neurologically within normal limits.

In contrast, children who manifest a sagittal cavus and are plantarflexed at the midfoot are rather common. Ballet is an example of an activity that can mold the midfoot into that attitude.

WHAT ASPECTS OF SHOE WEAR ARE IMPORTANT WHEN TREATING CHILDREN?

Although the assessment of shoes is important in both children and adults, children are hard on shoes and also go through them rapidly as a result of growth. Accordingly, good feedback can be obtained by assessing the shoes when new, and at intervals thereafter, because they tell a story in much same way that tire wear on a car aids the mechanic. In addition, as conveyed elsewhere in this article, children can at times be a challenge to performing meaningful gait assessment for a variety of reasons. Evaluation of shoe wear patterns can provide the clinician with useful information. In **Figs. 24** and **25**, note the asymmetry and location of wear at both the outer soles

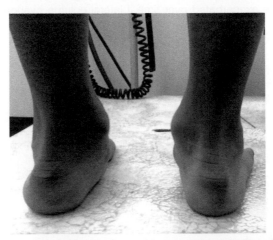

Fig. 22. Posterior view of the right hindfoot with angle of image directly posterior.

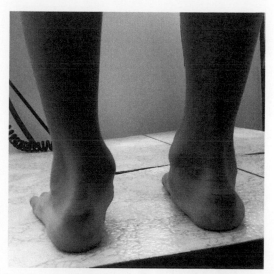

Fig. 23. Posterior view of the left hindfoot with angle of image directly posterior.

and the shoe counters. The right shoe demonstrates breakdown of the medial heel counter, excessive posteromedial heel wear and wear medial to the first metatarsal head. The left shoe demonstrates central-posterior heel wear, a relatively symmetric heel counter and wear centrally under the first metatarsal head. A differential can be generated by these findings alone (eg, unilateral torsional–rotational condition, limb length discrepancy, medial paresis on the right, asymmetric subtalar range, etc). Corroboration with biomechanical findings is essential; however, this element of the examination is not to be ignored.

Two further points bear mentioning. The first is that quality control in the manufacture of children's shoes is not always optimal, and the uppers are not always sewn perpendicular to the outer sole. As such, the shoe itself may be the cause of the abnormal wear, rather than the child. Accordingly, if the patient is already established, prudence suggests that new shoes first be approved by the clinician before they are

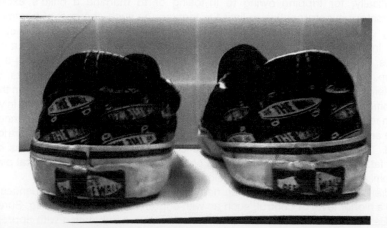

Fig. 24. Posterior view of left and right shoes.

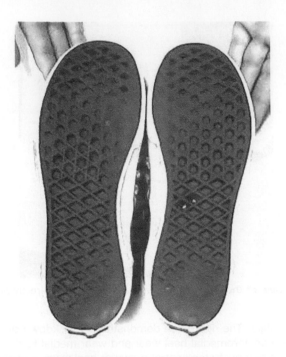

Fig. 25. Plantar view of left and right shoes.

used by the child. The second is that parents should be reminded to keep the shoes that the child has outgrown so that they can be evaluated by the clinician.

Orthotic Management

Although orthotics are a treatment modality rather than a part of the pediatric biomechanical assessment, they bear mentioning for several reasons. The choice to intervene in young children who are otherwise neurologically intact is undertaken, pragmatically, for tripping owing to in-toeing or to manage a child's excessive compensatory hyperpronation to limit the tripping. As such, the goal of treatment is, in many cases, supportive until the torsional or rotational condition corrects with growth. In these circumstances prefabricated foot orthoses, which come in a variety of styles, are usually adequate to fulfill this objective. Common to most is a deep heel cup, flat rearfoot post, or a combination of forefoot and rearfoot posts. When these elements are not present, deep medial and lateral flanges are included in the device. Some devices have all of these features. The inclusion of these elements in young children relates to the abundance of plantar flat in the heel area, which enhances the surface area to ground when barefooted, but also limits control when an orthotic is applied. The cupping effect of the device actually enhances the thickness of the plantar fat. As a result, the ability for the child to be controlled in the frontal plane is compromised if the orthosis is not designed to overcome it.

Children with hypotonia or other neurologic or neuromuscular influences may require a higher level of control, such as with supramalleolar orthoses (eg, Surestep, South Bend, IN), which are custom-fabricated and, in combination with appropriate shoes, can be useful in stabilizing gait without additional rigidity (**Fig. 26**).

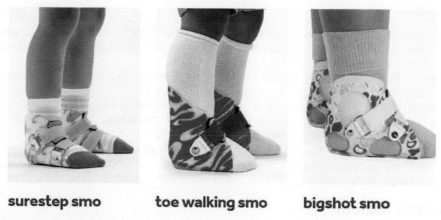

surestep smo   **toe walking smo**   **bigshot smo**

Fig. 26. Supramalleolar orthoses.

In either circumstance, the clinician should be aware that frequent assessment is required of the child with orthoses, owing to growth as well as the child's responsiveness to the effect of the orthosis on foot shape or position. In addition, remember that the shoe–orthosis combination delineates the degree of control, and not the orthosis alone.

FURTHER READINGS

MUSCLE TESTING IN CHILDREN

Escolar DM, Henricson EK, Mayhew J, et al. Clinical evaluator reliability for quantitative and manual muscle testing measures of strength in children. Muscle Nerve 2001;24(6):787–93.

Rose KJ, Burns J, Ryan MM, et al. Reliability of quantifying foot and ankle muscle strength in very young children. Muscle Nerve 2008;37(5):626–31.

Sloan C. Review of the reliability and validity of myometry with children [review]. Phys Occup Ther Pediatr 2002;22(2):79–93.

TORSION/ROTATION ASSESSMENT

Aird JJ, Hogg A, Rollinson P. Femoral torsion in patients with Blount's disease: a previously unrecognised component. J Bone Joint Surg Br 2009;91(10):1388–93.

Cusick BD, Stuberg WA. Assessment of lower-extremity alignment in the transverse plane: implications for management of children with neuromotor dysfunction [review]. Phys Ther 1992;72(1):3–15.

Harris E. The intoeing child: etiology, prognosis, and current treatment options [review]. Clin Podiatr Med Surg 2013;30(4):531–65.

Lincoln TL, Suen PW. Common rotational variations in children [review]. J Am Acad Orthop Surg 2003;11(5):312–20.

Sabharwal S, Lee J Jr, Zhao C. Multiplanar deformity analysis of untreated Blount disease. J Pediatr Orthop 2007;27(3):260–5.

EQUINUS

Gourdine-Shaw MC, Lamm BM, Herzenberg JE, et al. Equinus deformity in the pediatric patient: causes, evaluation, and management [review]. Clin Podiatr Med Surg 2010;27(1):25–42.

Greene WB. Cerebral palsy. Evaluation and management of equinus and equinovarus deformities [review]. Foot Ankle Clin 2000;5(2):265–80.

Tustin K, Patel A. A critical evaluation of the updated evidence for casting for equinus deformity in children with cerebral palsy [review]. Physiother Res Int 2017;22(1). https://doi.org/10.1002/pri.1646.

Wright J, Coggings D, Maizen C, et al. Reverse Ponseti-type treatment for children with congenital vertical talus: comparison between idiopathic and teratological patients. Bone Joint J 2014;96-B(2):274–8.

PEDIATRIC FLATFOOT

Ford SE, Scannell BP. Pediatric flatfoot: pearls and pitfalls [review]. Foot Ankle Clin 2017;22(3):643–56.

Hutchinson B. Pediatric metatarsus adductus and skewfoot deformity [review]. Clin Podiatr Med Surg 2010;27(1):93–104.

Kim HY, Shin HS, Ko JH, et al. Gait analysis of symptomatic Flatfoot in children: an observational study. Clin Orthop Surg 2017;9(3):363–73.

Rodriguez N, Volpe RG. Clinical diagnosis and assessment of the pediatric pes planovalgus deformity [review]. Clin Podiatr Med Surg 2010;27(1):43–58.

Zargarbashi RH, Bonaki HN, Zadegan SA, et al. Comparison of pediatric and general orthopedic surgeons' approaches in management of developmental dysplasia of the hip and flexible flatfoot: the road to clinical consensus. Arch Bone Jt Surg 2017;5(1):46–51.

METATARSUS ADDUCTUS

Williams CM, James AM, Tran T. Metatarsus adductus: development of a non-surgical treatment pathway [review]. J Paediatr Child Health 2013;49(9):E428–33.

GAIT DEVELOPMENT

Guffey K, Regier M, Mancinelli C, et al. Gait parameters associated with balance in healthy 2–4 year-old children. Gait Posture 2016;43:165–9.

Kim HY, Shin HS, Ko JH, et al. Gait analysis of symptomatic flatfoot in children: an observational study. Clin Orthop Surg 2017;9(3):363–73.

The Biomechanics of Diabetes Mellitus and Limb Preservation

Jonathan M. Labovitz, DPM[a],*, Dana Day, DPM[b,c]

KEYWORDS

- Diabetic foot • Biomechanics • Gait dysfunction amputation • Fall risk
- Foot pressure • Limb salvage

KEY POINTS

- Biomechanics of the diabetic foot are change over time owing to the disease process altering anatomic structures and musculoskeletal function.
- Static changes of the diabetic foot can be attributed to altered collagen, changes in muscle strength, soft tissue thickening, and eventually contractures and deformities.
- The dynamic changes seen in the lower extremity include modifications in gait, diminished postural stability, and increased sway.
- Clinically, the static and dynamic biomechanical changes alter plantar loading of the foot leading to ulceration and increase unsteadiness leading to a greater risk of falling.
- Amputations in the diabetic foot further change the biomechanics and overall function; however, amputations may sometimes still be better than salvage.

INTRODUCTION

The diabetic foot remains a significant health care issue that involves a collection of complex and intertwined conditions and ultimately leads to life-altering and life-shortening outcomes. It is easy to comprehend that these medical complexities with such damaging clinical outcomes result in a significant societal burden, ranging from the impact on families and caregivers to the costs to the health care system.

The medical conditions that collectively comprise the diabetic foot often revolve around diabetic peripheral neuropathy (DPN), peripheral arterial disease, infections, Charcot neuroarthropathy, and amputations. However, musculoskeletal changes alter

Disclosure Statement: The authors have nothing to disclose.
[a] Clinical Education and Graduate Services, College of Podiatric Medicine, Western University of Health Sciences, 309 East Second Street, Pomona, CA 91766, USA; [b] College of Podiatric Medicine, Western University of Health Sciences, 309 East Second Street, Pomona, CA 91766, USA; [c] Chino Valley Medical Center, Chino, CA 91710, USA
* Corresponding author.
E-mail address: jlabovitz@westernu.edu

Clin Podiatr Med Surg 37 (2020) 151–169
https://doi.org/10.1016/j.cpm.2019.08.011
0891-8422/20/© 2019 Elsevier Inc. All rights reserved.

podiatric.theclinics.com

the biomechanics of patients living with diabetes mellitus (DM). These changes impair daily function, making the biomechanical changes a principle underlying factor of most, if not all, of these commonly reported conditions.

This article discusses the static and dynamic biomechanical changes that impact the diabetic population. The clinical implications of the altered anatomic structures, gait, and the forces resulting from these changes are also reviewed. Last, the impact of lower extremity amputations on biomechanics and the associated downstream effects of the altered mechanics is discussed.

STATIC MUSCULOSKELETAL CHANGES IN DIABETES MELLITUS
Altered Collagen

DM impacts the musculoskeletal system in many ways. The array of intrinsic factors responsible for the changes stem from elevated blood sugar levels; however, there is no universally accepted explanation for the changes. Chronic hyperglycemia induces nonenzymatic glycosylation of proteins, which produces excessive advanced glycation end products and increased collagen cross-linking and decreasing susceptibility to collagen degradation within tendons.[1,2] Other studies report the altered local environment owing to high glucose concentrations encourages abnormal expression of type I collagen and decreases tenocyte proliferation, inhibits cell proliferation, induces cell apoptosis, and suppresses tendon-derived stem cell expression.[3,4]

The altered soft tissue microarchitecture results in structural abnormalities, mainly impacting the collagen of the tendons, ligaments, joint capsules, and the skin. The effects of glycolysis on periarticular collagen and tendons include thickened structures with decreased elasticity. For example, thickening of the Achilles and flexor hallucis longus tendons have been observed.[5,6]

Abnormal tendon collagen fibrils have been described in the Achilles tendon, which is one of the more well -described structures impacted by collagen abnormalities in DM. Using electron microscopy, Grant and colleagues[7] observed increased packing density of collagen fibrils, a decrease in fibrillar diameter, and abnormal fibril morphology. Impaired Achilles tendon collagen organization also includes increased fibril cross-linking and focal collagen degeneration, resulting in thickening of the Achilles tendon, leading to increased stiffness and decreased flexibility. Ultimately, the periarticular and tendon changes lead to limited joint mobility, which has downstream effects on gait.[5,7–10]

In fact, limited joint mobility is not exclusive to the ankle. In the foot reduced mobility of the subtalar joint, first metatarsal-phalangeal (MTP) joint and lesser MTP joints also occurs.[11–13] There is a decreased maximum knee joint angle in patients with diabetes regardless of neuropathy, although a higher knee angle has been reported at midstance.[14,15] Limited range of motion at the hip is more controversial. In patients with DPN, Gomes and associates[8] reported increased hip flexion as a compensatory mechanism for the limited joint mobility distally. Meanwhile, other studies demonstrate decreased hip flexion in patients with DPN compared with patients with DM without DPN.[16,17]

Muscle Mass and Strength

Hyperglycemia, obesity, insulin resistance, inflammatory cytokines, diabetes-related complications, and endocrine changes associated with diabetes accelerate reductions in muscle mass and strength, which are the 2 characteristics that define sarcopenia.[18–20] Patients with type 2 DM have been shown to have a 3-fold higher risk of sarcopenia compared with nondiabetic controls. This increased risk may result from defects in insulin signaling (which can decrease muscle synthesis) and malnutrition and disuse, all of which are associated with sarcopenia.[21] Clinically, sarcopenia results in frailty, which has diagnostic criteria including slower walking speed, diminished grip strength, and decreased physical inactivity. Frailty is associated with adverse outcomes such as increased falls, loss of independence, hospitalizations, and mortality.[19,20]

Loss of muscle strength and mass in the lower extremities are reported by many studies. Patients with DM experience a greater decline in strength and mass in the leg compared with nondiabetic controls.[22] Mueller and colleagues[23] identified a reduction in power, which they attributed to a decreased plantarflexory torque at the ankle. Meanwhile, Andersen and colleagues[24] reported decreased maximal isokinetic strength of the ankle and knee in patients with DPN and muscle atrophy. A greater decrease in maximal isokinetic strength was noted distally, with the ankle only exhibiting 59% of the strength of controls and the knee being 73% of controls. Overall muscle volume was diminished 32% with atrophy observed at the midleg (43%) and distal leg (65%) compared with controls. They concluded that muscle atrophy is also likely to explain the muscle weakness observed. However, a potential alternative explanation involves adipose tissue. According to a study by Tuttle and colleagues,[25] Patients with DPN had a higher calf intermuscular adipose tissue volume, which was associated with poor muscle strength and physical function.

In addition to muscle strength being decreased, contractions are delayed. Slower dorsiflexion contractile properties for evoked and voluntary contractions likely contribute to diminished muscle quality and slowed contraction.[26] As evidenced by delayed electromyography responses, deficits in the internal control mechanisms for motor control may also be responsible for ankle inefficiency and decreased shock absorption.[27] Muscles are also more easily fatigued, which Allen and colleagues[28] attribute to dysfunctional neuromuscular transmission.

Soft Tissue Thickening

In addition to tendons and periarticular structures, other soft tissues are altered in response to glycation end products from high glucose concentrations. Fibrosis, atrophy, and distal displacement of the plantar fat pad beneath the metatarsal heads occur in patients with DPN.[29,30] The heel fat pad increases in stiffness.[31] These changes decrease the shock absorption properties, preventing adequate cushioning of the metatarsal heads during stance and forefoot contact with the ground during gait. Significant thickening of the plantar fascia has been reported in patients with DM regardless of DPN presence compared with healthy controls.[5,6]

Thinning of the skin occurs early in DM. Hardening of the skin also occurs, commonly observed as excessive callus formation. This finding may occur later, because autonomic neuropathy is likely a contributing factor. Hardened skin is also commonly seen around active diabetic foot ulcers (DFUs), whereas those with a history of DFUs can experience increased stiffness and decreased tissue thickness.[32–34]

Contractures and Deformities

The soft tissue changes involving skin, ligaments, tendons, and other structures limit flexibility and joint motion, and may contribute to the contractures often observed in the diabetic foot. In addition to these limitations, motor neuropathy can cause a progressive atrophy of the intrinsic foot musculature. This atrophy contributes to the development of pes cavus and other deformities such as hallux valgus, digital contractures, and prominent plantar metatarsal heads.

One common contracture is hyperextension of the digits at the MTP joints. The hyperextension of the central MTP joints is frequently attributed to the intrinsic muscle atrophy. Although there is a decrease in muscle density owing to fatty infiltration of the intrinsic muscles in patients with diabetic neuropathy, this factor alone is unlikely to cause the contractures.[35] However, it is likely a contributing factor as Cheuy and colleagues[36] reported an association between patients with diabetes with decreased lean muscle volume and greater MTP joint hyperextension. The increased plantar fascia thickness in patients with diabetes, likely secondary to fibrosis of the tissues, may contribute to decreased joint mobility of the lesser MTP joints. Despite being a less common clinical entity, gross deformities such as a rocker bottom foot are known to occur after the remodeling phase of Charcot neuroarthropathy.

DYNAMIC MUSCULOSKELETAL CHANGES IN DIABETES MELLITUS

The importance of the static changes lies in their impact on the normal limb function. The resultant dynamic changes affect daily function, including altering gait, postural stability, and sway.

Gait

Gait characteristics have been described in multiple studies, systematic reviews, and meta-analyses. Many of the studies use a variety of systems to measure the kinetic and kinematic changes in patients with diabetes with and without DPN compared with healthy controls. The greatest changes in the altered kinematics of patients with DM involve DPN, although some changes are observed before the onset of sensory loss. These changes have been reported to impact the lower extremities, the pelvis, and spine (**Box 1**).

Patients with DPN can experience limited trunk mobility and postural deviations of the spine consisting of hyperlordosis and thoracic kyphosis. There can be an increased obliquity of the pelvis, including an anterior pelvic tilt.[15] Fernando and colleagues[37] found an increased anterior pelvic tilt during initial heel contact and greater pelvic obliquity in patients with an active DFU compared with nonhealthy controls and patients with DM in the absence of a DFU history. Positional changes at the knee include a lateral shift of the patella and external rotation, which rotates the foot, causing increased arch height.

During ambulation, the soft tissue stiffness alters joint function, and muscle weakness impacts eccentric contractions of the quadriceps and tibialis anterior decreasing joint stability, thus contributing to gait impairment and unsteadiness. A meta-analysis by Fernando and colleagues[38] showed that patients with diabetes and DPN exhibit longer overall stance time and higher plantar pressures. When evaluated as a percentage of the gait cycle, patients with DPN spent $61.07\% \pm 3.14\%$ of the gait cycle in stance compared with patients with DM ($59.7\% \pm 2.2\%$) and healthy controls

---

Box 1
Common compensatory gait strategies

- Wider base of support
- Shorter steps
- Slower gait
- Longer double support time

(59.4% ± 2.32%).[39] This meta-analysis did not determine significant slowing of walking speed, although most studies and a meta-analysis by Hazari and colleagues[14,23,40–42] reported significantly slower gait velocity.

Although most studies demonstrate altered gait in the DPN population, it is important to consider changes also occur in peripheral arterial disease. Pain-free and painful intermittent claudication (IC) alters time-based parameters, as well as kinetic and kinematic characteristics. The ischemic effects of IC during activity result in weakness of the propulsive muscles in the hip and calf posterior muscle groups, leading to failure supporting forward progression during gait. The muscle weakness accounts for the decreased hip extensor and ankle plantarflexor moments, which in turn reduces hip flexion and increases ankle plantarflexion after heel contact. Patients with IC adopt a more conservative gait with significantly more pronounced changes in painful IC, similar to the more pronounced changes in DPN, depending on the severity. Changes compared with healthy controls include slower velocity, decreased cadence and stride length, and increased double limb support. Painful IC also increases the time spent in stance phase.[43]

Postural Stability and Sway

Postural stability and sway require normal vestibular, visual, and somatosensory function. The instability in patients with DM most often stems from some combination of diminished sensory feedback, visual impairment, muscle weakness, and a lack of neuromuscular control of distal joints in neuropathic patients.[44] This unsteadiness typically occurs when ambulating, although a diminished feedback system or an inability to provide the proper stability can occur during stance or gait.

The vestibular and visual systems function to provide feedback allowing for postural correction to maintain stability. The vestibular system is sensitive to glycemic levels such that hyperglycemia causes an inability to detect anterior body translation.[45] The visual system, also negatively impacted by hyperglycemia, experiences diminished feedback when retinopathy is present.

Stability relies on muscle strength and perception of limb position, which occurs in response to feedback from cutaneous receptors, mechanoreceptors, and proprioceptive receptors within joint capsules and muscles. Postural stability becomes compromised when the somatosensory system experiences diminution or loss of tactile and proprioceptive sensation. An interruption of the normal afferent function of the tibial, sural, and deep peroneal nerves in ankle ligaments and joint capsule has been identified as a cause of deficient feedback.[46]

Sway is the back and forth movement of the body against the point of gravity during stance that occurs in response to postural muscle activity. Sway is likely impacted by the commonly observed changes in soft tissues, such as delayed reaction time, loss of muscle strength, and decrease in activity of the muscles required for postural stability.[47] The patient with DPN can have increased sway amplitude and velocity. Toosizadeh and colleagues[48] determined a higher rate of sway compared with controls when evaluating postural muscle control (local control), whereas involvement of central control, using sensory feedback, demonstrated a decreased rate of sway. Therefore, the lack of sensory feedback involving the somatosensory, vestibular, and visual systems can increase the rate of sway resulting in a high degree of instability. Yet there are adaptive strategies used to help adjust for the instability.

Although sway is increased in the presence of DPN, increased sway can occur in the absence of sensory loss. A significantly increased mediolateral sway during ambulation in patients with impaired glucose tolerance suggests altered sway and gait may be associated with impaired glucose tolerance and prediabetes.[49] Further support of glucose impairment as the foundation of increased instability may be seen in a study of pregabalin intervention. Improved gait stability did not occur when patients with painful DPN were given pregabalin. Instead, patients experienced increased variability in step length and gait speed, possibly increasing the fall risk.[50]

PLANTAR LOADING OF THE FOOT

In a foot with ideal structure and biomechanical function, one would expect a normal and equal distribution of pressure applied across the plantar aspect of the foot. When there is abnormal alignment or function, there are peak areas of pressure indicating excessive vertical forces applied to the foot during ground contact. The static and dynamic biomechanical changes involve variations in functional gait, reduced muscle activity and altered gait mechanics, which translates to increased plantar pressures.[51,52] Slower walking speed is one functional change that reduces plantar pressure. When walking speed was reduced from a normal rate of 1.19 m/s to a slow speed of 0.83 m/s, peak plantar pressure decreased at the heel (5%–18%), medial forefoot (9%–11%), and hallux (11%).[53]

Changes in muscle activity, such as eccentric control of tibialis anterior and early activation of ankle extensors, causes premature forefoot contact and subsequently increases the peak forefoot pressure and pressure time integral (PTI).[27,54] Patients with an active DFU also have impaired gait that causes a significantly longer duration of stance, and greater plantar pressures and PTI to the toes and midfoot compared with patients with DM without an ulcer and healthy controls. The plantar pressure and PTI remain increase in patients with a DFU at 6-month follow-up.[37,55]

The soft tissue changes decrease the ability of the tissues to function as a shock absorber; thus, pressure is poorly distributed and peak pressures occur. This is often the case with MTP joint contractures owing to distal displacement of the fat pad that often becomes fibrotic. Higher pressure to the heel in intermediate and late stages of DPN may be indicative of decreased shock absorption properties of the plantar heel fat pad.[27] Areas with excessive hyperkeratotic tissue are also sources of peak pressure, where treatment is supported by callus debridement resulting in lower plantar pressures.[56] The thickened plantar aponeurosis and Achilles tendon increases ground reactive forces.

Some postural changes specifically increase forefoot peak pressures with postural changes such as lordosis and increased anterior pelvic tilt, which cause increased pressures under the first metatarsal head.[15] Limited ankle dorsiflexion creates excessive loading of the foot during gait by preventing anterior progression of the tibia over the foot during the stance phase.[57] This leads to compensatory mechanisms such as early heel off, excessive subtalar joint protonation, and midtarsal protonation, which cause early and prolonged weight bearing on the forefoot.[13] Similarly, limited motion at the first MTP joint causes increased pressure secondary to premature loading of the hallux during propulsion.[58]

A meta-analysis evaluating the association between ankle equinus and plantar pressure in patients with DM demonstrated a significant but small effect.[59] Searle and colleagues[60] observed that patients with equinus were 2.2 times more likely to have high pressures compared with those without equinus and were significantly more likely to have at risk in-shoe forefoot pressures. They also significantly increased PTI ($P = .004$) and in-shoe PTIs ($P = .012$).

The location and magnitude of peak pressure varies based on foot position and comorbidities. Pes planus increases medial forefoot pressure, and obesity causes greater lateral forefoot pressure.[61] The decreased plantar surface seen with intrinsic foot muscle atrophy causing pes cavus also increases plantar loading.

To clarify the role of neuropathy in plantar pressure distribution, Sacco and colleagues[62] assessed differences in pressure based on the stage of neuropathy. Anterior migration of the pressures was observed beginning in early stage DPN with significantly higher peak pressures and PTI at the hallux and the forefoot area in intermediate and late stage neuropathy. They concluded that this finding may be linked to impaired toe off in the intermediate stage neuropathic patient and altered muscle activity for a portion of the increased PTI in the later stages.[54,62]

Shearing Forces

Much of the literature focuses on peak plantar pressures in the diabetic foot. Although it is critical to understand the vertical forces during gait, force vectors occur in 3 dimensions. Despite a longer stance phase increasing the contact area with the ground, active patients with a DFU experienced increased plantar pressure. This finding supports the notion that understanding shear forces is crucial.[37] The limited effort studying anterior to posterior and medial to lateral shearing forces may be due to the difficulty obtaining accurate measurements of these forces.[63] Additionally, both hardening and stiffness of the soft tissue increases shear forces.

Shearing forces are an important factor since shear force and peak pressure in patients with diabetes occurs in different locations, and peak pressure location is moderately correlated with plantar ulcers.[64,65] Yavuz and colleagues[65] studied shearing forces in patients with DPN compared with nondiabetic patients. They observed peak anterior-posterior shearing forces, and resultant shear magnitude was 33% ($P = .014$) and 31% ($P = .016$) greater in the diabetic neuropathy group. PTI (54%, $P = .013$), anterior-posterior shearing time integral (STI) (132%, $P<.05$) and resultant STI (61%, $P<.05$) were also significantly greater in the diabetic population. The elevated magnitudes of PTI and STI occurred despite the diabetic population having a 15% slower cadence, which may be partially explained by increased contact time during gait. The importance of shear forces is also supported by the greater magnitude of the increases in peak shearing forces and STI compared with that of peak pressure and PTI.

Regarding the location of shear forces, Yavuz and coworkers[64] reported they were located at the same site as peak pressure in only 20% of patients while they differed by more than 0.5 cm in 60% of patients.

THE CLINICAL IMPACT OF ALTERED BIOMECHANICS

Static and dynamic changes in the musculoskeletal system alter the functional mechanics of the foot, which subsequently increase ground reactive forces and shearing forces when standing and during ambulation. The added forces result in the damaging plantar loading implicated as a factor in the development of foot ulcers and potentially their associated limb- and life-threatening consequences.

Diabetic Foot Ulcers

Static and dynamic biomechanical impairment discussed earlier account for deformities and traumatic events, which are 2 components of the clinical triad that leads to DFU formation. Deformities and the resultant increase in pressure are well known to predispose patients to DFUs. Recently, in a multivariate analysis to determine ulcer risk, Farzy and associates[66] found patients with foot deformities had a significant likelihood of developing a DFU (odds ratio, 8.7; $P<.05$).[66]

Limited joint mobility increasing the plantar pressure increases trauma to the plantar foot predisposing the foot to a DFU.[12] Equinus prevalence is significantly greater in patients with an active DFU compared with patients with DM without an active DFU.[13] Diabetic populations with foot complications of DPN or a history of an ulcer or amputation also have increased prevalence of equinus, ranging from 72.4% to 91.0%.[67,68] In addition, Frykberg and associates[69] concluded that patients with DM with DPN are 2.8 times more likely to have equinus than those without DPN. Limited motion of other joints also impact DFU formation, such as the association between the first MTP joint and hallux ulcers.[11]

Muscle weakness, thickened soft tissue structures with decreased elasticity and flexibility can contribute to deformity formation. Increased maximum peak plantar pressure and changes in the pressure gradient are associated with ulcer formation. Pham and colleagues[70] determined a high maximum peak pressure, defined as equal to or greater than 6 K/cm^2, increased the risk of developing a DFU (odds ratio, 3.2; $P<.001$). However, there is some ambiguity regarding a threshold for developing a DFU and the best force measurement to use. Armstrong and colleagues[71] found that the increased peak plantar pressure was higher in the DFU group compared with controls. They concluded there was no optimal threshold because the best cut-off pressure was 70 N/cm^2 (sensitivity, 70.0%; specificity, 65.1%).[71] Meanwhile, Farzy and colleagues[66] reported 335 kPa (33.5 N/cm^2) as the optimal peak forefoot pressure threshold for ulcer risk based on sensitivity (60%), specificity (74%) and accuracy (71.8%). Hazari and coworkers[14,15] concluded that 60 N/cm^2 is the upper threshold for DFU development and most recently report a threshold of 60.38 N/cm^2.

When evaluating the measurement with the most clinical relevance, it is important to recognize that few studies correlate peak vertical pressure measurements and ulcer location.[72] Veves and colleagues[73] found that only 38% of ulcers were in the same location as the peak pressure and that the peak pressure location changed over the 30-month follow-up period in 59% of patients. This finding may be explained by considering peak shearing forces, which Yavuz and associates[64] found was at the same location as the peak pressure in 20% of patients, whereas they differed by more than 2.5 cm in 60% of patients. Giacomozzi and colleagues[5] reinforced the importance of shear forces when they found increased vertical ground reactive forces in patients with DPN compared with healthy controls, whereas increased vertical and mediolateral ground reactive forces were present in patients with DM with a history of foot ulcer. Both DPN and foot ulcer patients experienced increased maximum foot loading time in vertical, anteroposterior and mediolateral directions.

Lott and associates[74] investigated alternative metrics and concluded that the peak maximal shearing stress and peak pressure gradient are likely the most discriminatory measures, although the peak plantar pressure was also significant in patients with a history of DFU. These variables provide information on the distribution of the peak pressure and the internal stresses they cause, which may be detrimental to the tissues.[74] The peak maximal shear stress has been found to be higher and closer to the surface in the forefoot compared with the rearfoot.[75] Pressure gradients with excessive forefoot pressure in relation to rearfoot pressure are common in patients with a history of DFU.

Impact of Offloading

Offloading the foot during treatment of active DFUs supports the clinical consequences of increased plantar pressure. In a study of patients with active DFU, plantar pressures were higher in the active DFU participants compared with those with DM and no active DFU, which lead Fernando and colleagues[37] to conclude that this stresses the importance of offloading.

Offloading is used to treat active DFU and to prevent recurrence. Total contact casts and removable walkers have been shown to decrease plantar pressures more than other offloading devices, although therapeutic shoes with a rocker bottom sole with a molded insole also significantly decrease plantar pressures.[76] However, likely owing to nonadherence, removable walkers are equivalent to total contact casts once they are rendered nonremovable.[77–79]

Fall Risk

The medical literature is replete with studies documenting gait unsteadiness in DM. Altered gait, diminished postural stability, and increased sway result in poor balance while standing and when walking. Patients with DPN have both sensory and motor ability deficits, which impairs the efferent and afferent neural function crucial to stability. This loss of stability leads to a significantly greater risk of falls in the DPN population, which Cavanagh and coworkers[80] report as a 15 times greater risk in patients with DPN compared with patients with diabetes without DPN. Moreover, patients with painful DPN have a self-reported increased number of falls with subsequent hospitalizations.[81]

However, it is important to note that gait unsteadiness can precede sensory loss. Allet and colleagues[82] demonstrated that older patients with DM exhibit impaired balance and slower reaction time, and consequently have a higher risk of falling when compared with age-matched, control participants with DM. Meanwhile, nonbiomechanical factors also increase fall risk and may be independent of sensory loss because depression and cognitive deficits are associated with gait unsteadiness in patients living with DM.[83,84]

Increased variability in step width, wider and shorter step length, greater double limb support time, and slower speed are common compensatory mechanisms to provide stability during gait.[44,47,81,84–86] Patients with DPN often demonstrate these adaptive strategies when ambulating. The strategies are used to address the instability created by postural instability and the increased sway secondary to decreased ankle and knee strength, coupled with a greater muscular effort required to control the greater mediolateral distances between center of mass and center of pressure.[87,88] However, muscle weakness also slows gait velocity, so slower walking may not be exclusively compensatory.[84] More important, decreased survival is one consequence of a slowed gait.[89] In addition, reaction time to stop walking was found to be 2-fold higher in patients with diabetes without muscle weakness.[42] All of these adaptive gait strategies are likely the result of impaired vestibular, autonomic, and sensory nervous systems.[42,84]

Clinically, there are opportunities to minimize the fall risk by improving the somatosensory feedback and altered gait. A study comparing walking barefoot versus wearing shoes demonstrated decreased fall risk, likely owing to more pronounced changes in gait when barefoot. The study group wearing shoes exhibited significantly improved gait initiation velocity ($P<.005$), gait steady state velocity ($P<.01$), and the number of steps to achieve steady state gait velocity ($P = .05$).[86] Other investigators have reported that therapeutic shoes improve balance and, thus, decrease fall risk by increasing the tactile and proprioceptive mechanisms by improving feedback from cutaneous receptors and by reducing mediolateral motion of the center of mass during gait with appropriate footwear with a suitable arch support.[84] Thus, shoes may enhance the afferent somatosensory stimulus, helping to overcome the decreased joint mobility and increased joint stiffness that Kanade and colleagues[90] concluded augments falls in patients with DFUs.

Similar to DPN, peripheral arterial disease patients have an increased risk of falls. The reported decreased mobility and gait changes in patients with IC are similar to findings observed in patients with DPN, thus making them more prone to falling. Additionally, symptomatic peripheral arterial disease patients in the absence of IC, experience increased gait variability, which is known to increase instability and the risk of falling.[91]

THE IMPACT OF AMPUTATIONS

Although deformities such as digital contractures and hallux valgus can cause deviations in plantar pressure, so can lower extremity amputations (LEA). The removal of anatomic structures and inappropriate surgical technique when performing a LEA, which is often avoidable, alters the position and kinematics of the foot.

Deformities and Changes in Pressure

Partial foot amputations result in a change in the support surface. Considering that plantar pressure is the vertical ground reactive force divided by surface area, partial foot amputations increase plantar pressure.[92,93] Isolated or multiple digital amputations increase the load to the remainder of the foot, exacerbating the risk of complications secondary to vertical and shearing forces. Marks and associate[94] reported an increased risk of deformities to the remaining digits, which was also reported to occur in the second MTP joint and second and third digits after hallux amputation.[95] A hallux amputation is likely the most devastating digital LEA. A unilateral hallux LEA increases peak pressure and PTI under the first metatarsal head and lateral forefoot. The compensatory gait also results in increased pressure beneath the heel.[96,97]

Contractures and other deformities can occur owing to unopposed muscle function after resection or detachment of the opposing muscle or corresponding tendon. The unintended consequence of the unopposed forces results in foot deformity with increased forces to areas of the foot unable to accommodate the added pressure. Ray amputations also shift pressure to a smaller surface area, although they have potential for muscle imbalance as well. A first ray amputation can cause instability of the forefoot with decreased plantarflexion owing to loss of the tibialis anterior and/or peroneus longus. A fifth ray amputation can lead to forefoot adduction and an equinovarus deformity with loss of the peroneus brevis insertion.

Transmetatarsal amputations (TMA) are often implicated in altered biomechanics resulting in failed limb salvage. Iatrogenic causes include poor technique, which can result in abnormal pressure at the stump from improper residual length of the metatarsals (Fig. 1). Fig. 2 shows how an equinovarus foot owing to unopposed function of the gastrocnemius, soleus, tibialis anterior, and tibialis posterior muscles.[98] The increased plantar loading results from the equinovarus foot position and a lack of ankle dorsiflexion. A gastrocnemius or Achilles tendon lengthening (TAL) is commonly performed with a TMA to minimize the potential load to the forefoot and amputation stump. This approach has been successful in patients who underwent a TMA and developed an ulcer to the LEA stump. When a TAL was performed. there was a 91% healing rate of the ulcer.[99] However, Mueller and associates[100] demonstrated that the benefit of the TAL may persist clinically despite some benefits of the procedure being only temporary. They reported a decreased DFU recurrence after a TAL compared with a TCC at 2 years (38% vs 81%; $P = .002$) and an increased ankle dorsiflexion that remained at 7 months postoperatively; however, plantar flexor peak torque and peak plantar pressures of the forefoot during barefoot walking returned to baseline after 7 months.[100]

Gait is also altered after a TMA. Patients tend to have limited push-off power because there is decreased ankle plantarflexion power resulting in patients relying on pulling the leg forward at the hip. These changes are caused by decreased range

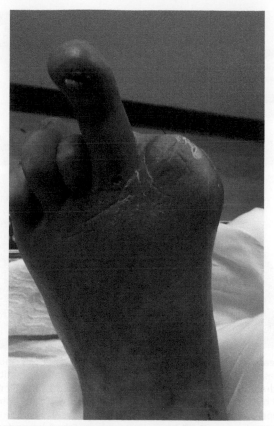

Fig. 1. An iatrogenic cause of abnormal loading of the forefoot secondary to inappropriate digital amputations resulting in a foot deformity prone to further complications. (*Courtesy of* S. Sadra, DPM, Pomona, CA.)

of motion excursion, peak moments, and peak ankle power at the ankle and decreased hip range of motion with an earlier onset of hip flexor moment.[101] More proximal minor amputations typically result in an increased risk of muscle imbalance with unopposed plantar flexors with further shortening of the lever arm and a smaller plantar surface area. These amputations are often poorly tolerated owing to decreased stability and poor push-off strength.[94]

Functional Amputations

A functional result is critical to maintaining independence, which impacts state of mind, quality of life and willingness to actively participate in self-care by controlling glycemic levels and preventing further complications. Mobility and ambulation are important factors in determining independence.

Partial foot amputations are considered successful limb salvage. Because these amputations are minor, which are defined as a LEA that preserves the ankle joint, we define success by the anatomic location. However, many LEAs are less than functional, leaving patients unable to preserve a sense of independence. An analysis of more than 400 first ray amputations concluded 1 of 5 first ray LEA require a more proximal amputation to achieve a durable, weight bearing extremity.[102] Faglia and colleagues[103] studies Chopart amputations and found 59.6% of patients had delayed

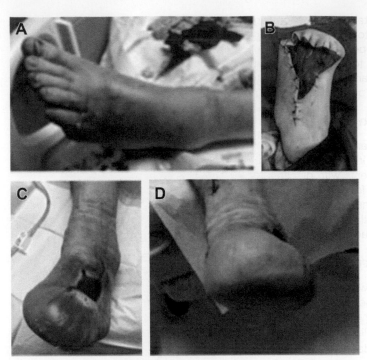

Fig. 2. (*A*) A 52-year-old man diagnosed with diabetic ketoacidosis and sepsis presented with necrotizing fasciitis of the left foot. (*B*) A transmetatarsal amputation was performed with incision and drainage of the more proximal soft tissues. (*C*) After 5 months, the patient was nearly healed but had a residual equinovarus deformity. (*D*) At 7 months, the patient returned to the operating room for tendon balancing to decrease the increased load to the plantar and lateral forefoot. This goal was accomplished by performing an Achilles tendon lengthening, anterior tibialis tendon transfer, and tenotomy of the tibialis posterior tendon.

weight bearing owing to a postoperative ulcer or went on to major amputation, thus demonstrating the potential for limited function. Partial LEA as distal as the tarsometatarsal joint affect general temporal-spatial ground reactive forces, ankle kinetics, and plantar pressure during gait.[104]

Larsson compared minor and major amputations finding the number healed and re-amputation rates were equal between the groups. However, minor LEA patients had a significantly greater percentage of patients who returned to walking capacity (70% vs 19%) and returned to independent living (93% vs 61%) than a major LEA. Major LEA had lower rehabilitation potential and higher mortality rates.[105]

However, a below-knee amputation with a proper prosthesis can be functional. Brown and coworkers[106] reported that 75% of patients undergoing a blow-knee amputation were ambulatory with a prosthesis and concluded that a longer stump may decrease the capacity to ambulate owing to instability associated with a longer stump. Functional limb salvage also depends on cardiovascular reserves. Most patients with diabetes have decreased cardiovascular reserves and the more proximal the LEA, the greater the oxygen consumption.[107,108] Goktepe and colleagues[109] attributed the greater energy expenditure to the gait asymmetry resulting from impaired ankle function and foot leverage, the high complication rates and challenges fitting prostheses.

Ultimately, when performing limb salvage procedures we must consider preserving the limb to allow for the greatest opportunity to maintain a functional limb for mobility and independence. This requires an attempt to restore normal biomechanics with attention to improving sagittal and transverse plane alignment.[110] This focus on the biomechanics of the procedure potentially maximizes the ability to stand, walk, and maintain postural stability and daily function.

SUMMARY

Biomechanical changes in the patient living with diabetes can significantly impact function, independence, quality of life, and mortality. Therefore, it is important to evaluate patients with diabetes for biomechanical changes to preserve both static and dynamic factors that change the gait and loading to the foot to decrease the risk of ulcerations and preserve balance and postural stability to prevent falls. Equally important are the changes associated with limb salvage. These biomechanical changes must be addressed to prevent deformities and potentially loss of function or life.

REFERENCES

1. Brownlee M, Vlassara H, Cerami A. Nonenzymatic glycosylation and the pathogenesis of diabetic complications. Ann Intern Med 1984;101(4):527–37.
2. Somai P, Vogelgesang S. Limited joint mobility in diabetes mellitus: the clinical implications. J Musculoskelet Med 2011;28(4):118–24.
3. Ueda Y, Inui A, Mifune Y, et al. The effects of high glucose condition on rat tenocytes *in vitro* and rat Achilles tendon *in vivo*. Bone Joint Res 2018;7(5): 362–72.
4. Lin YC, Li YJ, Rui YF, et al. The effects of high glucose on tendon-derived stem cells: implications of the pathogenesis of diabetic tendon disorders. Oncotarget 2017;8(11):17518–28.
5. Giacomozzi C, D'Ambrogi E, Uccioli L, et al. Does the thickening of the Achilles tendon and plantar fascia contribute to the alteration of diabetic foot loading? Clin Biomech 2005;20(5):532–9.
6. Bolton NR, Smith KE, Pilgram TK, et al. Computed tomography to visualize and quantify the plantar aponeurosis and flexor hallucis longus tendon in the diabetic foot. Clin Biomech 2005;20(5):540–6.
7. Grant WP, Sullivan R, Sonenshine DE, et al. Electron microscopic investigation of the effects of diabetes mellitus on the Achilles tendon. J Foot Ankle Surg 1997; 36(4):272–8.
8. Gomes AA, Onodera AN, Otuzi ME, et al. Electromyography and kinematic changes of gait cycle at different cadences in diabetic neuropathic individuals. Muscle Nerve 2011;44(2):258–68.
9. Guney A, Vatansever F, Karaman I, et al. Biomechanical properties of Achilles tendon in diabetic vs. non-diabetic patients. Exp Clin Endocrinol Diabetes 2015;123(7):428–32.
10. Turner DE, Helliwell PS, Burton AK, et al. The relationship between passive range of motion and range of motion during gait and plantar pressure measurements. Diabet Med 2007;24(11):1240–6.
11. Birke JA, Franks BD, Foto JG. First ray joint limitation, pressure, and ulceration of the first metatarsal head in diabetes mellitus. Foot Ankle Int 1995;16(5):277–84.
12. Delbridge L, Perry P, Marr S, et al. Limited joint mobility in the diabetic foot: relationship to neuropathic ulceration. Diabet Med 1988;5(4):333–7.

13. Mueller MJ, Diamond JE, Delitto A, et al. Insensitivity, limited joint mobility, and plantar ulcers in patients with diabetes mellitus. Phys Ther 1989;69(6):453–9.

14. Hazari A, Maiya AG, Shivashankara KN, et al. Kinetics and kinematics of diabetic foot of type 2 diabetes mellitus with and without peripheral neuropathy: a systematic review and meta-analysis. Springerplus 2016;5(1):1819.

15. Hazari A, Maiya AG, Shivashankara KN. Foot kinetic and kinematic profile in type 2 diabetes mellitus with peripheral neuropathy. J Am Podiatr Med Assoc 2019;109(1):36–49.

16. Raspovic A. Gait characteristics of people with diabetes-related peripheral neuropathy, with and without a history of ulceration. Gait Posture 2013;38(4):723–8.

17. Yavuzer G, Yetkin I, Toruner FB, et al. Gait deviations of patients with diabetes mellitus: looking beyond peripheral neuropathy. Eura Medicophys 2006;42(2): 127–33.

18. Morley JE, Malmstrom TK, Rodriguez-Manas L, et al. Frailty, sarcopenia and diabetes. J Am Med Dir Assoc 2014;15(12):853–9.

19. Umegaki H. Sarcopenia and diabetes: hyperglycemia is a risk factor for age-associated muscle mass and functional reduction. J Diabetes Investig 2015; 6(6):623–4.

20. Jang HC. Sarcopenia, frailty, and diabetes in older adults. Diabetes Metab J 2016;40(3):182–9.

21. Kim TN, Park MS, Yang SJ, et al. Prevalence and determinant factors of sarcopenia in patients with type 2 diabetes: the Korean Sarcopenic Obesity Study (KSOS). Diabetes Care 2010;33(7):1497–9.

22. Park SW, Goodpaster BH, Strotmeyer ES, et al. Accelerated loss of skeletal muscle strength in older adults with type 2 diabetes: the health, aging, and body composition study. Diabetes Care 2007;30(6):1507–12.

23. Mueller MJ, Minor SD, Sahrmann SA, et al. Differences in the gait characteristics of patients with diabetes and peripheral neuropathy compared with age-matched controls. Phys Ther 1994;74(4):299–308.

24. Andersen H, Gadeberg PC, Brock B, et al. Muscular atrophy in diabetic neuropathy: a stereological magnetic resonance imaging study. Diabetologia 1997; 40(9):1062–9.

25. Tuttle LJ, Sinacore DR, Cade WT, et al. Lower physical activity is associated with higher intermuscular adipose tissue in people with type 2 diabetes and peripheral neuropathy. Phys Ther 2011;91(6):923–30.

26. Allen MD, Major B, Kimpinski K, et al. Skeletal muscle morphology and contractile function in relation to muscle denervation in diabetic neuropathy. J Appl Physiol (1985) 2014;116(5):545–52.

27. Sacco IC, Amadio AC. Influence of diabetic neuropathy on the behavior of electromyographic and sensorial responses in treadmill gait. Clin Biomech (Bristol, Avon) 2003;18(5):426–34.

28. Allen MD, Kimpinski K, Doherty TJ, et al. Decreased muscle endurance associated with diabetic neuropathy may be attributed partially to neuromuscular transmission failure. J Appl Physiol (1985) 2015;118(8):1014–22.

29. Brash PD, Foster J, Vennart W, et al. Magnetic resonance imaging techniques demonstrate soft tissue damage in the diabetic foot. Diabet Med 1999;16(1): 55–61.

30. Bus SA, Maas M, Cavanagh PR, et al. Plantar fat pad displacement in neuropathic diabetic patients with toes deformity: a magnetic resonance imaging study. Diabetes Care 2004;27(10):2376–81.

31. Cheung YY, Doyley M, Miller TB, et al. Magnetic resonance elastography of the plantar fat pads: preliminary study in diabetic patients and asymptomatic volunteers. J Comput Assist Tomogr 2006;30(2):321–6.
32. Charanya G, Patil KM, Narayanamurthy VB, et al. Effect of foot sole hardness, thickness and footwear on forefoot pressure distribution parameters in diabetic neuropathy. Proc Inst Mech Eng H 2004;218(6):431–43.
33. Klaesner JW, Hastings MK, Zou D, et al. Plantar tissue stiffness in patients with diabetes and peripheral neuropathy. Arch Phys Med Rehabil 2002;83(12): 1796–801.
34. Piagessi A, Romanelli M, Schipani E, et al. Hardness of plantar skin in diabetic neuropathic feet. J Diabetes Complications 1999;13(3):129–34.
35. Robertson DD, Mueller MJ, Smith KE, et al. Structural changes in the forefoot in individuals with diabetes and a prior plantar ulcer. J Bone Joint Surg Am 2002; 84(8):1395–404.
36. Cheuy VA, Hastings MK, Commean PK, et al. Intrinsic foot muscle deterioration is associated with metatarsophalangeal joint angle in people with diabetes and neuropathy. Clin Biomech 2013;28(9–10):1055–60.
37. Fernando ME, Crowther RG, Lazzarini PA, et al. Plantar pressures are higher in cases with diabetic foot ulcers compared to controls despite a longer stance phase duration. BMC Endocr Disord 2016;16(1):51.
38. Fernando M, Crowther R, Lazzarini P, et al. Biomechanical characteristics of peripheral neuropathy: systematic review and meta-analysis from gait cycle, muscle activity and barefoot plantar pressure. Clin Biomech 2013;28(8):831–45.
39. Sawacha Z, Spolaor F, Guameri G, et al. Abnormal muscle activation during gait in diabetes patients with and without neuropathy. Gait Posture 2012;35(1): 101–5.
40. Sawacha Z, Gabriella G, Cristoferi G, et al. Diabetic gait and posture abnormalities: a biomechanical investigation through three dimensional gait analysis. Clin Biomech 2009;24(9):722–8.
41. Allet L, Armand S, Golay A, et al. Gait characteristics of diabetic patients: a systematic review. Diabetes Metab Res Rev 2008;24(3):173–91.
42. Petrofsky J, Lee S, Bweir S. Gait characteristics in people with type 2 diabetes mellitus. Eur J Appl Physiol (1985) 2005;93(5–6):640–7.
43. Chen SJ, Pipinos I, Johanning J, et al. Bilateral claudication results in alterations in the gait biomechanics at the hip and ankle joints. J Biomech 2008;41(11): 2506–14.
44. Menz HB, Lord SR, St George R, et al. Walking stability and sensorimotor function in older people with diabetic peripheral neuropathy. Arch Phys Med Rehabil 2004;85(2):245–52.
45. Hamada SM, Debrky HM. Monitoring of motor function affection and postural sway in patients with type 2 diabetes mellitus. Egypt J Ear Nose Throat Allied Sci 2014;15(3):241–5.
46. Chitra J, Shetty SS. Screening of proprioception of the ankle joint in patients with diabetic neuropathy–an observational study. Int J Ther Rehabil Res 2015;4(4): 104–7.
47. Mustafa A, Justine M, Mustafah NM, et al. Postural control and gait performance in the diabetic peripheral neuropathy: a systematic review. Biomed Res Int 2016;2016:9305025.
48. Toosizadeh N, Mohler J, Armstrong DG, et al. The influence of diabetic peripheral neuropathy on local postural muscle and central sensory feedback balance control. PLoS One 2015;10(8):e0135255.

49. Almurdhi MM, Brown SJ, Bowling FL, et al. Altered walking strategy and increased unsteadiness in participants with impaired glucose tolerance and type 2 diabetes relates to small-fibre neuropathy but not vitamin D deficiency. Diabet Med 2017;34(6):839–45.
50. Karmakar S, Rashidian H, Chan C, et al. Investigating the role of neuropathic pain relief in decreasing gait variability in diabetes mellitus patients with neuropathic pain: a randomized, double-blind crossover trial. J Neuroeng Rehabil 2014;11:125.
51. Andersen H. Motor dysfunction in diabetes. Diabetes Metab Res Rev 2012; 28(Suppl 1):89–92.
52. van Deursen R. Mechanical loading and off-loading of the plantar surface of the diabetic foot. Clin Infect Dis 2004;39(Suppl 2):S87–91.
53. Rosenbaum D, Hautmann S, Gold M, et al. Effects of walking speed on plantar pressure patterns and hindfoot angular motion. Gait Posture 1994;2:191–7.
54. Kwon OY, Minor SD, Maluf KS, et al. Comparison of muscle activity during walking in subjects with and without diabetic neuropathy. Gait Posture 2003; 18(1):105–13.
55. Fernando ME, Crowther RG, Lazzarini PA, et al. Plantar pressures are elevated in people with longstanding diabetes-related foot ulcers during follow-up. PLoS One 2017;12(8):e0181916.
56. Murray HJ, Young MJ, Hollis S, et al. The association between callus formation, high pressures and neuropathy in diabetic foot ulceration. Diabet Med 1996; 13(11):979–82.
57. Lavery LA, Armstrong DG, Boulton AJ, et al. Ankle equinus deformity and its relationship to high plantar pressure in a large population with diabetes mellitus. J Am Podiatr Med Assoc 2002;92(9):479–82.
58. Fernando DJ, Masson EA, Veves A, et al. Relationship of limited joint mobility to abnormal foot pressures and diabetic foot ulceration. Diabetes Care 1991; 14(1):8–11.
59. Searle A, Spink MJ, Ho A, et al. Association between ankle equinus and plantar pressures in people with diabetes: a systematic review and meta-analysis. Clin Biomech 2017;43:8–14.
60. Searle A, Spink MJ, Chuter VH. Prevalence of ankle equinus and correlation with foot plantar pressures in people with diabetes. Clin Biomech 2018;60:39–44.
61. Tang UH, Zugner R, Lisovskaja V, et al. Foot deformities, function in the lower extremities, and plantar pressure in patients with diabetes at high risk to develop foot ulcers. Diabet Foot Ankle 2015;6:27593.
62. Sacco IC, Hamamoto AN, Tonicelli LM, et al. Abnormalities of plantar pressure distribution in early, intermediate, and late stages of diabetic neuropathy. Gait Posture 2014;40(4):570–4.
63. Perry JE, Hall JO, Davis BL. Simultaneous measurement of plantar pressure and shear forces in diabetic individuals. Gait Posture 2002;15(1):101–7.
64. Yavuz M, Erdemir A, Botek G, et al. Peak plantar pressure and shear locations: relevance to diabetic patients. Diabetes Care 2007;30(10):2643–5.
65. Yavuz M, Tajaddini A, Botek G, et al. Temporal changes of plantar shear distribution: relevance to diabetic patients. J Biomech 2008;41(3):556–9.
66. Farzy OA, Arafa AI, Wakeel MA, et al. Plantar pressure as a risk assessment tool for diabetic foot ulceration in Egyptian patients with diabetes. Clin Med Insights Endocrinol Diabetes 2014;7:31–9.
67. Boffeli TJ, Bean JK, Natwick JR. Biomechanical abnormalities and ulcers of the great toe in patients with diabetes. J Foot Ankle Surg 2002;41(6):359–64.

68. Van Gils CC, Roeder B. The effect of ankle equinus upon the diabetic foot. Clin Podiatr Med Surg 2002;19(3):391–409.

69. Frykberg RG, Bowen J, Hall J, et al. Prevalence of equinus in diabetic versus non-diabetic patients. J Am Podiatr Med Assoc 2012;102(2):84–8.

70. Pham H, Armstrong DG, Harvey C, et al. Screening techniques to identify people at high risk for diabetic foot ulceration: a prospective multicenter trial. Diabetes Care 2000;23(5):606–11.

71. Armstrong DG, Peters EJ, Athanasiou KA, et al. Is there a critical level of plantar foot pressure to identify patients at risk for neuropathic foot ulceration? J Foot Ankle Surg 1998;37(4):303–7.

72. Wrobel JS, Najafi B. Diabetic Foot biomechanics and gait dysfunction. J Diabetes Sci Technol 2010;4(4):833–45.

73. Veves A, Murray HJ, Young MJ, et al. The risk of foot ulceration in diabetic patients with high foot pressure: a prospective study. Diabetologia 1992;35(7): 660–3.

74. Lott DJ, Zou D, Mueller MJ. Pressure gradient and subsurface shear stress on the neuropathic forefoot. Clin Biomech 2008;23(3):342–8.

75. Zou D, Mueller MJ, Lott DJ. Effect of peak pressure and pressure gradient on subsurface shear stresses in the neuropathic foot. J Biomech 2007;40(4): 883–90.

76. Bus SA, Valk GD, van Deursen RW, et al. The effectiveness of footwear and off-loading interventions to prevent and heal foot ulcers and reduce plantar pressure in diabetes: a systematic review. Diabetes Metab Res Rev 2008; 24(Suppl 1):S162–80.

77. Armstrong DG, Lavery LA, Wu S, et al. Evaluation of removable and irremovable cast walkers in the healing of diabetic foot wounds. Diabetes Care 2005;28(3): 551–4.

78. Katz IA, Harlan A, Miranda-Palma B, et al. A randomized trial of two irremovable off-loading devices in the management of plantar neuropathic diabetic foot ulcers. Diabetes Care 2005;28(3):555–9.

79. Piagessi A, Macchiarini S, Rizzo L, et al. An off-the-shelf instant contact casting device for the management of diabetic foot ulcers: a randomized prospective trial versus traditional fiberglass cast. Diabetes Care 2007;30(3):586–90.

80. Cavanagh PR, Derr JA, Ulbrecht JS, et al. Problems with gait and posture in neuropathic patients with insulin dependent diabetes mellitus. Diabet Med 1992;9(5):469–74.

81. Lalli P, Chan A, Garven A, et al. Increased gait variability in diabetes mellitus patients with neuropathic pain. J Diabetes Complications 2013;27(3):248–54.

82. Allet L, Armand S, de Bie RA, et al. The gait and balance of patients with diabetes can be improved: a randomised controlled trial. Diabetologia 2010; 53(3):458–66.

83. Vileikyte L, Leventhal H, Gonzalez JS, et al. Diabetic peripheral neuropathy and depressive symptoms: the association revisited. Diabetes Care 2005;28(10): 2378–83.

84. Brach JS, Talkowski JB, Strotmeyer ES, et al. Diabetes mellitus and gait dysfunction: possible explanatory factors. Phys Ther 2008;88(11):1365–74.

85. Dingwell JB, Cusumano JP, Sternad D, et al. Slower speeds in patients with diabetic neuropathy lead to improved local dynamic stability of continuous overground walking. J Biomech 2000;33(10):1269–77.

86. Najafi B, Khan T, Fleischer A, et al. The impact of footwear and walking distance on gait stability in diabetic patients with peripheral neuropathy. J Am Podiatr Med Assoc 2013;103(3):165–73.

87. Andreassen CS, Jakobsen J, Andersen H. Muscle weakness: a progressive late complication in diabetic distal symmetrical polyneuropathy. Diabetes 2006; 55(3):806–12.

88. Brown SJ, Handsaker JC, Bowling FL, et al. Diabetic peripheral neuropathy compromises balance during daily activities. Diabetes Care 2015;38(6): 1116–22.

89. Studenski S, Perera S, Patel K, et al. Gait speed and survival in older adults. JAMA 2011;305(1):50–8.

90. Kanade RV, Van Deursen RW, Harding KG, et al. Investigation of standing balance in patients with diabetic neuropathy at different stages of foot complications. Clin Biomech 2008;23(9):1183–91.

91. Myers SA, Johanning JM, Sterigou N, et al. Gait variability is altered in patients with peripheral arterial disease. J Vasc Surg 2009;49(4):924–31.

92. Garbalosa JC, Cavanagh PR, Wu G, et al. Foot function in diabetic patients after partial amputation. Foot Ankle Int 1996;17(1):43–8.

93. Armstrong DG, Lavery LA. Plantar pressures are higher in diabetic patients following partial foot amputation. Ostomy Wound Manage 1998;44(3):30–6.

94. Marks RM, Long JT, Extern EL. Gait abnormality following amputation in diabetic patients. Foot Ankle Clin 2010;15(3):501–7.

95. Quebedeaux TL, Lavery LA, Lavery DC. The development of foot deformities and ulcers after great toe amputation in diabetes. Diabetes Care 1996;19(2): 165–7.

96. Motawea M, Kyrillos F, Hanafy A, et al. Impact of big toe amputation on foot biomechanics. Int J Adv Res 2015;3(12):1224–8.

97. Lavery LA, Lavery DC, Quebedeax-Farnham TL. Increased foot pressures after great toe amputation in diabetes. Diabetes Care 1995;18(11):1460–2.

98. Pollard J, Hamilton GA, Rush S, et al. Mortality and morbidity after transmetatarsal amputation: retrospective review of 101 cases. J Foot Ankle Surg 2006; 45(2):91–7.

99. Barry DC, Sabacinski KA, Habershaw GM, et al. Tendo Achilles procedures for chronic ulcerations in diabetic patients with transmetatarsal amputations. J Am Podiatr Med Assoc 1993;83(2):96–100.

100. Mueller MJ, Sinacore DR, Hastings MK, et al. Effect of Achilles tendon lengthening on neuropathic plantar ulcers. A randomized clinical trial. J Bone Joint Surg Am 2003;85(8):1436–45.

101. Mueller MJ, Salsich GB, Bastian AJ. Differences in the gait characteristics of people with diabetes and transmetatarsal amputation compared with age-matched controls. Gait & Posture 1998;7(3):200–6.

102. Borkosky SL, Roukis TS. Incidence of re-amputation following partial first ray amputation associated with diabetes mellitus and peripheral sensory neuropathy: a systematic review. Diabet Foot Ankle 2012;3. https://doi.org/10.3402/dfa. v3i0.12169.

103. Faglia E, Clerici G, Frykberg R, et al. Outcomes of Chopart amputation in a tertiary referral diabetic Foot clinic: data from a consecutive series of 83 hospitalized patients. J Foot Ankle Surg 2016;55(2):230–4.

104. Dillion MP, Barker TM. Preservation of residual foot length in partial foot amputation: a biomechanical analysis. Foot Ankle Int 2006;27(2):110–6.

105. Larsson J, Agardh CD, Apelqvist J, et al. Long-term prognosis after healed amputation in patients with diabetes. Clin Orthop Relat Res 1998;350:149–58.
106. Brown BJ, Iorio ML, Klement M, et al. Outcomes after 294 transtibial amputations with the posterior myocutaneous flap. Int J Low Extrem Wounds 2014; 13(1):33–40.
107. Waters RL, Perry J, Antonelli D, et al. Energy cost of walking of amputees: the influence of level of amputation. J Bone Joint Surg Am 1976;58(1):42–6.
108. Pinzur MS, Gold J, Schwartz D, et al. Energy demands for walking in dysvascular amputees as related to the level of amputation. Orthopedics 1992;15(9): 1033–6.
109. Goktepe AS, Cakir B, Yilmaz B, et al. Energy expenditure of walking with prostheses: comparison of three amputation levels. Prosthet Orthot Int 2010; 34(1):31–6.
110. Attinger C, Venturi M, Kim K, et al. Maximizing length and optimizing biomechanics in foot amputations by avoiding cookbook recipes for amputation. Semin Vasc Surg 2003;16(1):44–66.

Lower Extremity Biomechanical Examination of Athletes

Patrick A. DeHeer, DPM FFPM RCPS (Glasg)[a,b,c,]*, Ankit Desai, DPM[a],
Joseph H. Altepeter, DPM[a]

KEYWORDS

- Lower extremity • Biomechanical • Overuse injury • Athlete

KEY POINTS

- A comprehensive lower extremity examination is a critical examination component for any type of injury in an athlete but should also be part of a preseason or preventive care program.
- Identification and treatment of biomechanical abnormalities and association with evidence-based risk factors for lower extremity disorders can be incorporated to potentially reduce risk or prevent acute and chronic injuries.

Thomas Edison said, "The doctor of the future will give no medication but will interest his patients in the care of the human frame, diet and in the cause and prevention of disease."[1] Preventive medicine is preferred to therapeutic medicine. The external pressures associated with caring for athletic patients magnifies the importance of preventive care. The role of prevention in athletes is centered on a comprehensive biomechanical examination combined with an understanding of the risk factors for common overuse or traumatic injuries.

Disclosures: Dr P.A. DeHeer is the Residency Director of St. Vincent Hospital Podiatry Program in Indianapolis, IN. He is a Fellow of the American College of Foot and Ankle Surgeons, a Fellow of the American Society of Podiatric Surgeons, a Fellow of the American College of Foot and Ankle Pediatrics, a Fellow of the Royal College of Physicians and Surgeons of Glasgow Fellowship of Faculty of Podiatric Medicine, and a Diplomate of the American Board of Podiatric Surgery. Dr A. Desai is a preceptor at Hoosier Foot & Ankle, Indianapolis, IN. Dr J.H. Altepeter is a podiatry resident at St. Vincent Hospital Podiatry Residency, Indianapolis, IN.
[a] Surgery, St. Vincent Hospital, 2001 W 86th St, Indianapolis, IN 46260, USA; [b] Surgery, Johnson Memorial Hospital, Franklin, 1125 W Jefferson St, Franklin, IN 46131, USA; [c] Department of Podiatric Medicine and Radiology, Rosalind Franklin University of Medicine and Science, 3333 Green Bay Rd, North Chicago, IL 60064, USA
* Corresponding author. Hoosier Foot and Ankle, 1159 West Jefferson Street Suite 204, Franklin, IN 46131.
E-mail address: padeheer@sbcglobal.net

Clin Podiatr Med Surg 37 (2020) 171–194
https://doi.org/10.1016/j.cpm.2019.08.012
0891-8422/20/© 2019 Elsevier Inc. All rights reserved.

The ever-changing landscape of clinical lower extremity biomechanical theories creates confusion. Root biomechanical theory served as the unquestioned foundation of lower extremity biomechanics for decades.[2] Alternative biomechanical theories emerged to challenge the Root theories, although many of these biomechanical theories do not align with surgical evidence-based medicine.[3–9] Described here is Root theory. It is based on core principles, albeit still applicable to surgical intervention, but seems to be fading for biomechanical treatment of lower extremity disorders.[2]

1. A normal foot type is defined and used to classify abnormal foot types based on the following:
   a. The bisector of the calcaneus is in line or parallel with the bisector of the lower one-third of the leg
   b. The plane of all 5 metatarsal heads is perpendicular to the calcaneal bisector
   c. Normal foot alignment occurs only when the subtalar joint (STJ) is positioned in neutral and the midtarsal joint fully locked between midstance and heel-off
2. Intrinsic foot deformities leading to abnormal motion (compensation) resulting in pathologic situations include:
   a. Forefoot varus
   b. Forefoot valgus
   c. Rearfoot varus
3. Cornerstones of the management paradigm are:
   a. Determine whether an intrinsic deformity is present
   b. Measure the amount of the deformity using a goniometer
   c. Cast the patient's foot to capture the degree of deformity in a plaster model
   d. Construct a functional foot orthosis consisting of wedges or posts, positioning either the forefoot and/or rearfoot, depending on the foot deformity, into a STJ neutral position while locking the midtarsal joints
   e. The functional foot orthoses would act to prevent abnormal or excessive foot motion (compensation)

The arguments against Root theory center on its inaccuracies associated with clinical measurement of deformities and its reliance on the calcaneal bisection as a reference point.[8–12] Jarvis and colleagues[11] argued that neutral calcaneal stance position is irrelevant for symptom-free feet. The findings showed no relation between historically defined deformities and foot kinematics.[11] They claim that Root's study had numerous flaws and far-reaching conclusions.[13] As such, surgical and radiological research on deformity correction and optimal alignment are dichotomous to these emerging biomechanical theories.[14–30]

One of the leading biomechanical theories emerging to supplant Root is the tissue stress approach.[30] The tissue stress theory is based on the location and function of the patient's injured tissue and an orthotic is designed to reduce the stress while improving function.[13] A foundational belief of medicine, especially sports medicine, is preventive care. Risk factors for overuse and acute injuries in athletes are well documented, and many are based on Root biomechanical theory. Meanwhile, tissue stress theory does not lend itself to preventive care, whereas Root does.

This article not only documents evidence-based risk factors for acute and overuse injuries linked to abnormal findings but, more importantly, provides an accessible review for a comprehensive lower extremity biomechanical examination for athletes. The ultimate goal for lower extremity health care providers is to keep athletes on the field or court, instead of on the injured reserve list. To do so, clinicians must know what risk factors to look for, and how to correctly find them before even considering treatment options.

RISK FACTORS FOR LOWER EXTREMITY INJURIES IN ATHLETES

The association between an accurate biomechanical examination and uncovering risk factors for both overuse and acute injuries in the athlete is critical for sports medicine lower extremity health care providers. At a minimum, the physician recognizing and addressing the biomechanical abnormality may potentially prevent an injury that could have led to a subsequently missed competition. Diagnosing to the best of their abilities, providers can prevent tragic career-ending injuries in athletes, who may have otherwise faced a worst-case scenario had it not been for the well-versed clinician (**Boxes 1–18**).

BIOMECHANICAL EXAMINATION OF THE LOWER EXTREMITY

A systematic examination of the lower extremity is critical to fully assess the athlete.[31,144] Although some of the clinical examination techniques of the foot and ankle in particular have been questioned in the literature, as mentioned earlier, there is still merit in evaluating things such as forefoot deformity and rearfoot position because they are linked to risk factors for injury. Proper evaluation techniques and experience help improve intrarater reliability. Further research may also lead to more reliable clinical examination techniques. These advances may be in improved equinus evaluation, or sequential replacement of clinical examination with largely radiographic imaging, such as hindfoot alignment views or weight-bearing computed tomography scans. Nonetheless, as of the publication of this article, the examination techniques listed later are still well recognized among lower extremity health care providers.

HIP EXAMINATION
Active Range-of-motion Tests

- Abduction
  - Patient standing, spreads legs apart to maximum comfortable limit
  - At minimum, each extremity should be 45° away from midline
- Adduction
  - Patient standing, crosses legs, tested leg in front of the weight-bearing leg, to maximum comfortable limit
  - At minimum, each extremity cross must at least 20° past midline
- Flexion
  - Patient supine, draws a knee as close as comfortably possible to the chest without bending the back
  - Each hip joint should allow approximately 135° of flexion

---

Box 1
Nonspecific lower extremity overuse injury

- Hip abductor weakness[32]
- Hip external rotator weakness[32]
- Increased quadriceps strength[33]
- Inflexibility of hamstrings[34]
- Knee stiffness[35]
- Rearfoot varus[34]
- Increased pronation excursion[36]

Box 2
Nonspecific lower extremity stress fracture

- Limb length discrepancy[37–39]
- Excessive hip external rotation[39]
- Genu valgum[39]
- Decreased calf girth[38,39]
- Equinus[39]
- Rearfoot varus[38,40]
- High medial longitudinal arch[37,39]
- Pes planus[39]
- Forefoot varus[37,39]
- Increased loading rate[41]

- Extension
  - Patient sitting
  - With back straight, arms crossed across chest, patient rises from chair

Passive Range-of-motion Tests (Note: Examiner Must Stabilize Patient's Pelvis Differently for Each Maneuver)

- Flexion (Thomas test) ∼ 120°
  - Patient supine
  - Examiner stabilizes pelvis by placing own hand under the patient's lumbar spine
  - Examiner flexes patient's hip joint
    - Patient's lumbar spine flattens on examiner's hand under patient
    - Patient's remaining hip flexion is now isolated to hip joint only
- Extension ∼ 30°
  - Patient prone
  - Examiner stabilizes pelvis by placing own arm over the patient's iliac crest and lower lumbar spine
  - Patient slightly bends knees to relax hamstring muscles
  - Examiner places examiner's other hand under patient's thigh, and lifts extremity upward
- Abduction ∼ 45°
  - Patient supine
  - Examiner stabilizes pelvis by placing own forearm across the abdomen and own hand on the opposite anterior superior iliac spine (ASIS)
  - Examiner then holds 1 ankle and gently abducts the extremity to maximum comfortable limit
- Adduction ∼ 20°
  - Patient supine
  - Examiner stabilizes pelvis by placing own forearm across the abdomen and own hand on the opposite ASIS

Box 3
Groin injury

- Hip adductor weakness[42]

Box 4
Femoral neck stress fracture

- Restricted rearfoot inversion[43]

---

   o Examiner holds 1 ankle and gently guides the leg over the opposite extremity to maximum comfortable limit
- Internal rotation ~35° versus external rotation ~45°
   o Standard method
      ▪ Patient supine, extremities extended
      ▪ Examiner stands at foot of examination table, holds patient's ankles just proximal to the malleoli
      ▪ Examiner rotates legs from the malleoli internally and externally, using the proximal end of the patella as a guideline to evaluate range of rotation
   o Alternative method
      ▪ Patient sitting up, hips flexed, knees bent, legs hanging over the end of the table
      ▪ Examiner stabilizes patient's thigh to ensure femur is not pulled from side to side during test
      ▪ Examiner grips the distal leg and rotates the whole limb externally and internally using the tibia and fibula as levers
      ▪ Thus, tibia acts as a useful pointer to exaggerate any slight differences of rotation

Muscle Strength Testing

- Flexors
   o Patient sitting up near edge of examination table, legs dangling
   o Examiner stabilizes pelvis by placing own hand over the patient's ipsilateral iliac crest
   o Patient raises thigh greater than 90° from table level to isolate iliopsoas muscle
   o Examiner gently places own other hand at patient's distal thigh and offers resistance until patient reaches maximum strength grade possible
- Extensors
   o Patient lies prone, flexes knee joint to relax hamstring muscle, and thereby isolates the gluteus maximus muscle
   o Examiner places own forearm over the iliac crests to stabilize the patient's pelvis
   o Patient raises thigh from the table
   o Examiner gently places own other hand onto the posterior aspect of the thigh, just proximal to the knee joint, and offers resistance until patient reaches maximum strength grade possible

---

Box 5
Trochanteric bursitis

- Gluteus medius inflexibility[44]
- Lateral pelvic tilt[44]

> **Box 6**
> **Hamstring injury**
>
> - Poor lumbar posture[45,46]
> - Restricted hip extension[47,48]
> - Decreased hamstring/quadriceps strength ratio[45,46,49–52]
> - Shortened hamstring length[45]
> - Inflexibility of hamstrings[45,46,53,54]
> - Hamstring weakness[55]
> - Side-to-side hamstring strength imbalance[51,52,56]
> - Equinus[48]

- Abductors
  - Standard method
    - Patient lying on a lateral side, supporting extremity below is bent for balance, pelvis is stacked, and spine is neutral
    - Examiner stabilizes pelvis by using the first web space of own hand to grasp the superior rim of the iliac crest
    - Patient raises tested extremity up into abduction
    - Examiner gently places own other hand at the distal-lateral aspect of the extremity, just proximal to the ankle, and offers resistance until patient reaches maximum strength grade possible
  - Alternative method
    - Patient supine, extremities already abducted 20°
    - Examiner gently places own hand on the distal-lateral aspect of each extremity, just proximal to the ankle, and offers resistance until patient reaches maximum strength grade possible to simultaneously test hip abductors
- Adductors
  - Standard method
    - Patient lying on a lateral side, the supporting extremity below is bent for balance, pelvis is stacked, and spine is neutral
    - Patient raises the tested extremity up into abduction
    - Examiner gently places own other hand at the distal-medial aspect of the extremity, just proximal to the ankle
    - As patient actively attempts to adduct extremity back to midline, examiner offers resistance until patient reaches maximum strength grade possible

> **Box 7**
> **Iliotibial band syndrome**
>
> - Excessive ipsilateral trunk flexion[57]
> - Excessive hip adduction[57–60]
> - Hip abductor weakness[58,61,62]
> - Genu varum[58]
> - Decreased knee flexion angle at foot strike[63]
> - Excessive internal rotation of tibia on femur[57–59,61,64]

Box 8
Knee disorder, including patellofemoral pain syndrome and anterior cruciate ligament injury

- Impaired core proprioception[65,66]
- Restricted hip extension[47]
- Excessive hip abduction[67]
- Increased hip external rotation strength[68]
- Excessive hip internal rotation[68]
- Quadriceps weakness[68]
- Hamstring weakness[68–70]
- Reduced knee flexion[68,71]
- Excessive knee abduction[58,68–72]
- Equinus[73]
- Increased navicular drop[68]
- Landing in-toe[67]

   ○ Alternative method
     ▪ Patient supine, both extremities already abducted 20°
     ▪ Examiner gently places their own other hand at the distal-medial aspect of the extremity, just proximal to each ankle
     ▪ As patient actively attempts to adduct extremities back to midline together, examiner offers resistance until patient reaches maximum strength grade possible to simultaneously test hip adductors

Leg Length Discrepancy

- True (structural) leg length discrepancy
  ○ Patient supine, legs in neutral position
  ○ Examiner begins measurement at the slight concavity just below the ASIS.
    ▪ Measure distance from ASIS to respective medial malleolus of each extremity
    ▪ Unequal distances between these fixed points verify that one extremity is shorter than the other: a true (structural) leg length discrepancy

---

Box 9
Patellar tendinopathy

- Hip extensor weakness[58]
- Reduced hip internal rotation[74]
- Hip external rotation weakness[74]
- Inflexibility of hamstrings[75]
- Inflexibility of quadriceps[75]
- Genu varum[76]
- Genu valgum[76]
- Forefoot varus[74]

Box 10
Pes anserinus bursitis

- Inflexibility of hamstrings and sartorius[44]
- Genu valgum[44,77]
- Excessive foot pronation[44]

- Differentiating tibial versus femoral discrepancy in true (structural) leg length discrepancy
  - Patient supine, knees flexed to 90° but feet flat on examination table
  - Examiner evaluates for knee-to-knee relationship
    - If one knee appears higher than the other, the contralateral tibia is longer
    - If one knee projects further anteriorly than the other, the femur of that extremity is longer
- Apparent (functional) leg length discrepancy
  - First, examiner must rule out a true leg length discrepancy
  - Patient supine, legs in neutral position
  - Examiner measures from umbilicus to medial malleoli of the ankle of each extremity
    - Unequal distances here, but true leg length measurements being equal, indicate apparent (functional) leg length discrepancy

Ober Test for Contraction of the Iliotibial Band

This test is shown in **Fig. 1.**

- Patient in lateral recumbent position, involved leg uppermost
  - Neutral spine
  - Stacked (perpendicular) pelvis
- Examiner places their own hand (index on ASIS, thumb on posterior superior iliac spine, web space braces iliac crest) to stabilize patient's pelvis
- Examiner uses own other hand to cup patient's anterior-medial knee and own forearm to support patient's medial leg with knee at 90°
- Examiner abducts and lifts extremity posteriorly into slight hip extension, but keeping knee flexed at 90°
- Examiner gently releases abducted leg to observe passive thigh movement
  - Thigh drops into adduction indicates normal iliotibial (IT) band (negative Ober test)
  - Thigh remains abducted indicates contracture of IT band (positive Ober test)

Box 11
Medial tibial stress syndrome

- Limited hip mobility[78]
- Tibial varum[79]
- Equinus[78,79,108]
- Pronated foot type[80–82]
- Medial deviation of forefoot pressure[83]

Box 12
Exercise-related leg pain

- Excessive foot pronation[36,84]

KNEE EXAMINATION
Collateral Ligament Stability

- Medial collateral ligament (MCL)
  - Patient supine, examination knee is unlocked just enough to avoid full knee extension
  - Examiner's lateral hand placed against the knee so thenar eminence is against the fibular head
  - Examiner's medial hand secures the ankle
  - Examiner's lateral hand pushes medially against the knee and laterally against the ankle to open up the knee joint medially (thereby applying a valgus stress)
    - A medial gap indicates insufficient MCL
- Lateral collateral ligament (LCL)
  - Patient supine, examination knee is unlocked just enough to avoid full knee extension
  - Examiner's medial hand placed against the knee so thenar eminence is against the medial tibial condyle
  - Examiner's lateral hand secures the ankle
  - Examiner's medial hand pushes laterally against the knee and medially against the ankle to open up the knee joint laterally (thereby applying a varus stress)
    - A lateral gap indicates insufficient LCL

Cruciate Ligament Stability

- Anterior cruciate ligament (ACL); **Fig. 2**
  - Patient supine, knees flexed to 90°, feet flat on table.
  - Examiner stabilizes feet by sitting on them
  - Examiner cups own hands around the patient's knee
    - Fingers around medial and lateral hamstrings, thumbs on medial and lateral joint lines

---

Box 13
Achilles tendinopathy

- Reduced knee flexion during gait[85]
- Plantarflexor weakness[86–88]
- Equinus[43,108,109]
- Excessive ankle joint dorsiflexion[87]
- Rearfoot valgus[40]
- Excessive rearfoot inversion[43]
- Excessive rearfoot eversion[85]
- Low medial longitudinal arch[89]
- High medial longitudinal arch[40]
- High braking force[89]

Box 14
Retrocalcaneal bursitis

- Equinus[44]
- Rearfoot varus[44]

  - ○ Examiner forcibly pulls the tibia anteriorly
    - ■ If tibia slides distinctly under the femur, that is considered a positive anterior draw sign, indicating possible tear of ACL
- Posterior cruciate ligament (PCL)
  - ○ Patient supine, knees flexed to 90°, feet flat on table
  - ○ Examiner stabilizes feet by sitting on them
  - ○ Examiner cups own hands around the patient's knee
    - ■ Fingers around medial and lateral hamstrings, thumbs on medial and lateral joint lines
  - ○ Examiner forcibly pushes the tibia posteriorly
    - ■ If tibia slides distinctly under the femur, that is considered a positive posterior draw sign, indicating possible tear of PCL

Active Range-of-motion Tests

- Flexion
  - ○ Ask patient to squat in a deep knee bend
    - ■ Both knees should bend symmetrically
- Extension
  - ○ Instruct the patient to stand up from the squatting position
- Internal and external rotation
  - ○ Instruct patient to rotate foot medially and laterally

Passive Range-of-Motion Tests

- Flexion ~ 135°
  - ○ Patient supine
  - ○ Examiner grasps patient's leg just proximal to the ankle and places another hand in the popliteal fossa to act as a fulcrum and to unlock the knee

---

Box 15
Chronic ankle instability

- Poor postural control[90]
- Poor coordination[91]
- Hip extension weakness[92]
- Faster reaction of tibialis anterior and gastrocnemius during sudden inversion[91]
- Equinus[91]
- Decreased dorsiflexion/plantarflexion strength ratio[91,93]
- Increased eversion/inversion strength ratio[93]
- Poor inversion proprioception[94]
- Excessive first metatarsophalangeal joint dorsiflexion[94]
- Laterally deviated center of pressure at initial contact[95]

Box 16
Posterior tibial tendinopathy

- Limb length discrepancy[96]
- Genu valgum[96]
- Equinus[96]
- Excessive rearfoot pronation[39,97,98]
- Pes planus[96]

- o Examiner flexes the leg to maximum limit comfortable and notes specifically the distance between the heel and buttock
- Extension ~ 0°
  - o Patient supine
  - o Examiner keeps hold of patient's leg just proximal to the ankle with other hand in the popliteal fossa to act as a fulcrum
  - o Examiner extends the leg from flexion to maximum limit comfortable and looks specifically for a smooth arc and a healthy level of minor hyperextension
- Internal rotation ~10° versus external rotation ~10°
  - o Patient supine
  - o Examiner places own hand on patient's thigh just above the knee to stabilize the femur and grasps the heel with remaining free hand
  - o Examiner rotates the tibia internally and then externally, palpating the tibial tuberosity for reference of motion

Muscle Strength Testing

- Extension
  - o Patient sitting up with legs dangling from examination table
  - o Examiner stabilizes femur by placing 1 hand just above the knee
  - o Patient fully extends knee
  - o Once fully extended, examiner offers resistance to extension just proximal to the ankle joint
- Flexion
  - o Patient prone
  - o Examiner stabilizes thigh just proximal to knee joint
  - o Patient flexes knee to perpendicular to examination table
  - o Examiner then grasps ankle and provides resistance to patient's flexion.
- Internal and external
  - o Not possible to isolate muscles for manual muscle testing here; can be evaluated with flexion by internally and externally rotating leg

---

Box 17
Tarsal and metatarsal stress fracture

- Excessive rearfoot inversion[43]
- Rearfoot varus[99]
- Metatarsus adductus[106,107]

Box 18
Plantar fasciitis

- Inflexibility of hamstrings[100]
- Genu varum[40]
- Equinus[39,77,100,101,103–105]
- Cavus foot type[39,40,78]
- Low medial longitudinal arch[100,102]
- High vertical ground reactive forces[102]

McMurray Test

- Patient supine, with legs flat in neutral position
- Examiner holds the patient's heel with 1 hand
- Examiner places other hand on patient's knee joint and flexes the knee to full flexion
  - Fingers touching the medial joint line
  - Thumb and thenar eminence against the lateral joint line
- Examiner rotates the leg internally and externally to loosen the knee joint while sequentially stressing the knee to evaluate for any click indicating possible posterior meniscal tear
  - Examiner pulls on the medial side of the knee to apply a varus stress to the lateral side of the joint while rotating the leg internally
  - Maintain the varus stress and internal rotation and extend the leg slowly while palpating the lateral joint line
    - A click indicates a possible posterior tear of the lateral meniscus
  - Flex the knee back to complete flexion
  - Push on the lateral side to apply a valgus stress to the medial side of the joint while rotating the leg externally
  - Maintain the valgus stress and external rotation and extend the leg slowly while palpating the medial joint line
    - A click indicates a possible posterior tear of the medial meniscus

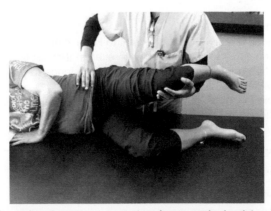

Fig. 1. Ober test for IT band contraction. Patient has a stacked pelvis and neutral spine in lateral recumbent position. Examiner stabilizes pelvis, abducts and lifts from bent knee, observes passive thigh movement.

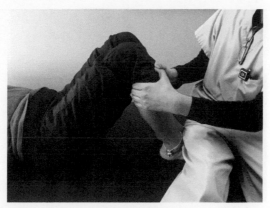

Fig. 2. ACL test. Patient is supine with knees bent. Examiner stabilizes feet, forcibly pulls tibia anteriorly, observes for tibial slide forward.

Apley Compression Test

- The Apley test is a compression/grinding test
- Patient is prone with examination leg flexed 90°
- Examiner gently kneels on the back of the patient's thigh to stabilize it, while leaning hard on the heel to compress the medial and lateral menisci between the tibia and femur
- Next, examiner rotates the tibia internally and externally on the femur while maintaining firm compression
  - If this elicits pain, there is probably meniscal damage
    - Ensure patient describes the exact location of the pain
      - Pain medially suggests medial meniscus tear
      - Pain laterally suggests lateral meniscus tear

Apley Distraction Test

- Used to distinguish meniscal versus ligamentous disorders
- Test should logically follow Apley compression test
- Patient is still prone
- Examiner is still kneeling on patient's posterior thigh for stabilization
- Examiner applies traction to the leg while rotating the tibia internally and externally on the femur
  - Pain reports pain, indicates ligamentous damage
  - No pain, meniscus alone was likely torn

ANKLE EXAMINATION
Ankle Dorsifexion Examination Testing for Equinus

Ankle dorsifexion examination testing for equinus[17,18,110] is shown in **Fig. 3**.

- Patient is supine on examination table, the foot is supinated
- Goniometer center is placed at lateral ankle joint, with one arm along lateral leg bisection of the fibula, the other on lateral margin of foot
- With knee extended and the foot maximally supinated, examiner dorsiflexes the ankle to firm end range of motion; greater than 5° dorsiflexion is considered normal
- With knee flexed and the foot maximally supinated, examiner dorsiflexes the ankle to end range of motion; greater than 10° dorsiflexion is considered normal

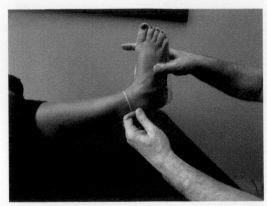

Fig. 3. Ankle dorsiflexion for equinus. Patient knee fully extended. Examiner supinates STJ while dorsiflexing ankle joint, observes for range of motion via goniometer.

Active Range-of-motion Ankle Tests

- Ankle plantarflexion
  - ○ Instruct patient to walk on toes
- Ankle dorsiflexion
  - ○ Instruct patient to walk on heels

Muscle Strength Testing

- Tibialis anterior
  - ○ Instruct the patient to invert and dorsiflex the foot as examiner provides resistance
- Extensor hallucis longus
  - ○ Instruct patient to dorsiflex the hallux as examiner provides resistance that is distal to interphalangeal joint
- Extensor digitorum longus
  - ○ Instruct patient to dorsiflex the digits as examiner provides individual resistance to each lesser digit with thumb
- Peroneus longus and brevis
  - ○ Instruct the patient to plantarflex and evert the foot against resistance that the examiner places at head of fifth metatarsal
- Gastrocnemius and soleus
  - ○ As a functional test, instruct patient to hop on the ball of one foot, 1 at a time
  - ○ In a supine position, instruct the supine patient to plantarflex the balls of the feet against resistance
- Flexor hallucis longus
  - ○ Instruct patient to plantarflex hallux against resistance
- Flexor digitorum longus
  - ○ Instruct the patient to curl the toes against resistance
- Tibialis posterior
  - ○ Instruct the patient to plantarflex and invert the foot against resistance.

Joint Stability Testing

- Isolated anterior talofibular ligament (ATFL) test
  - ○ Examiner turns the patient's foot into plantarflexion and then inversion
  - ○ Pain on inversion indicates ATFL injury

- Anterior draw test of ankle (**Fig. 4**)
  - Patient seated with legs dangling comfortably, feet slightly in plantarflexion
  - Examiner pushes on distal-anterior tibia posteriorly with 1 hand, but grips calcaneus in palm of other hand and pulls anteriorly to draw calcaneus with talus forward
  - Any distinct anterior slide of the talus under the ankle mortise is considered a positive drawer sign
- Lateral ankle instability test (talar tilt test, **Fig. 5**)
  - Examiner places the ankle in anatomic position and then inverts the calcaneus
    - If talus gaps and rocks in ankle mortise:
      - Both ATFL and calcaneal fibular ligament (CFL) are injured
- If there is just pain with inversion but no gapping:
  - The CFL is likely injured
- Medial ankle instability test
- Examiner stabilizes patient's leg by grasping the tibia with 1 hand and the calcaneus with the other
- Evert the patient's foot
- Gross gapping at ankle mortise: medial deltoid ligament injury

FOOT EXAMINATION
Passive Range-of-motion Tests

- First-ray position ~10 mm (**Fig. 6**)
  - Patient supine, with STJ placed in neutral position
  - Examiner grasps the second through fifth metatarsal heads, cupping them collectively between thumb and index finger
    - Tip: nail plate of examiner's thumb should be parallel to plane of metatarsals
  - With the other hand, examiner holds the first metatarsal head in a similar fashion
  - Evenly load the foot
  - Examiner moves first metatarsal dorsally and plantarly and records motion
    - Tip: total first ray range of motion (ROM) should be roughly 10 mm
  - Examiner also records first metatarsal excursion relative to second metatarsal
    - Tip: this provides objective information to diagnose a dorsiflexed or plantar-flexed first ray deformity

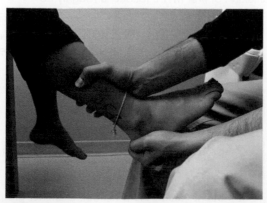

Fig. 4. Anterior drawer. Patient leg dangling comfortably. Examiner pushes tibia posteriorly but pulls heel with talus anteriorly, observing for anterior talar slide.

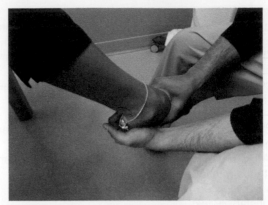

Fig. 5. Talar tilt (isolating ATFL). Examiner plantarflexes then inverts foot, observing for pain indicating ATFL injury. When ankle is in anatomic neutral position, it is inverted to check for both ATFL and calcaneal fibular ligament injury.

Tip: Measurements Going Forward Require a Goniometer

First metatarsal phalangeal joint (MTPJ) Dorsiflexion ROM.

- Metatarsal heads unloaded
  - Patient supine
  - Examiner places goniometer arms
    - Distal arm: medial aspect of the proximal phalanx
    - Proximal arm: medial bisection of the first metatarsal
  - Examiner dorsiflexes the first MTPJ
    - Tip: dorsiflexion of first MTPJ unloaded is roughly 70°
- Metatarsal heads loaded
  - Patient supine
  - Examiner places goniometer arms
    - Distal arm: medial aspect of proximal phalanx
    - Proximal arm: plantar surface of the foot
  - Examiner applies pressure to plantar surface of first metatarsal head, and dorsiflexes the first MTPJ
    - Tip: dorsiflexion of first MTPJ loaded is roughly 20°

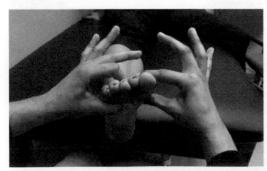

Fig. 6. First-ray range of motion. Patient STJ is neutral. Examiner grasps second through fifth metatarsals in one hand, and first metatarsal head in other hand, loads the foot, then puts first ray through ROM and observes.

Table 1
Gait examination

Checkpoint	Joint	Sign/Symptom	Cause
Stance Phase			
Heel strike	Foot	Antalgic gait from	Plantar fasciitis, heel pain
	Knee	Patient pushing knee into extension with a hand	Unstable knee gait caused by weak quadriceps
Forefoot loading	Foot	Foot slap	Weak or nonfunctioning anterior leg (extensor) muscle group
Midstance	Foot	Painful plantar metatarsal head calluses	Fallen transverse arch
		Pain when walking on uneven ground	Rigid pes planus or subtalar joint arthritis
		Painful hyperkeratosis on dorsum of toes	Dorsal toe corns rubbing against shoe as toes begin to grip the ground
	Knee	Unstable knee	Weak quadriceps unable to stabilize traditionally unlocked knee
	Hip	Gluteus medius lurch (patient lurching toward weaker side to place the center of gravity over the hip joint)	Weakened gluteus medius muscle on involved side
		Gluteus maximus lurch (patient must thrust the thorax posteriorly to maintain hip extension)	Weak gluteus maximus
Push-off	Foot	Pain on lateral side of the foot	DJD of first MTPJ makes patient unable to hyperextend the first MTPJ, thus patient is forced to push off from the naturally less robust lateral side of the foot
		Pain on plantar metatarsal head	Plantar calluses developed because of a plantarflexed metatarsal head
	Knee	Calcaneal (flat-footed) gait	Weakness of gastrocnemius, soleus, and/or flexor hallucis longus
Swing Phase			
Acceleration	Foot	Ankle not held in neutral	Weak ankle dorsiflexors
	Knee	Extremity not bent short enough to clear the ground	Knee did not reach maximum degree of flexion between toe-off and midswing, approximately 65°
	Hip	Exaggerated anterior pelvis rotation to provide forward thrust for the leg	Weak quadriceps unable to contract hip just before toe-off
Midswing	Foot	Shoe scrape	Weak ankle dorsiflexors
		Compensatory steppage gait	Weak ankle dorsiflexors require patient to flex the hip excessively to bend the knee so foot may clear the ground

(continued on next page)

Table 1 (continued)			
Checkpoint	Joint	Sign/Symptom	Cause
Deceleration	Knee	Back knee gait	Forced knee hyperextension from weak hamstrings
		Thickening of heel pad	Heel strike may be excessively harsh because of weak hamstrings not able to slow down swing in controlled manner

Abbreviation: DJD, degenerative joint disease.

Subtalar Joint Neutral Position

- Patient prone with distal one-third of leg hanging off edge of table
- Examiner marks with pen:
  - Heel bisection
  - Leg bisection
- Examiner palpates medial and lateral aspect of talar head as STJ is moved from an everted position to an inverted position
- When talar head feels equally prominent on medial and lateral sides, examiner adds a loading force to the forefoot and the ankle joint is dorsiflexed to 90°
- Examiner compares heel bisection with leg bisection with goniometer

Forefoot Position

- Patient prone, with STJ placed in neutral position and midtarsal joint locked, or fully pronated
- Examiner applies a dorsiflexion loading force to the forefoot at metatarsal heads
  - Tip: do not manipulate MTPJs during this procedure
- Using a goniometer, compare the plane of the metatarsal heads on the planar surface of the foot with heel bisection
  - Measure first through fifth metatarsal head angle to heel bisection
    - Tip: ideally, result should be perpendicular
  - Measure second through fifth metatarsal head angle to heel bisection

Resting Calcaneal Stance Position

- Patient standing in angle and base of gait
- Examiner measures heel bisection to weight-bearing surface with goniometer

Neutral Calcaneal Stance Position

- Patient standing, with STJ placed in neutral position
- Examiner measures heel bisection to weight-bearing surface with goniometer

GAIT EXAMINATION

Table 1 highlights components of each phase of the gait cycle to be evaluated, along with symptoms to be aware of that may clue to an underlying cause.

Summary

A comprehensive lower extremity examination on an athlete is a critical examination component for any type of injury but should also be part of a preseason or preventive care program (see **Table 1**). Identification and treatment of biomechanical abnormalities and association with evidence-based risk factors for lower extremity disorders can be incorporated to potentially reduce risk or prevent acute and chronic injuries.

REFERENCES

1. Available at: https://www.azquotes.com/quote/347519?ref5preventive-medicine. Accessed April 8, 2019.
2. Root ML, Orien WP, Weed JH. Biomechanical examination of the foot. Los Angeles (CA): Clinical Biomechanics Corp; 1971.
3. Sobel E, Levitz SJ, Caselli MA, et al. Reevaluation of the relaxed calcaneal stance position. Reliability and normal values in children and adults. J Am Podiatr Med Assoc 1999;89(5):258–64.
4. Payne CB. The past, present, and future of podiatric biomechanics. J Am Podiatr Med Assoc 1998;88(2):53–63.
5. Nigg BM. The role of impact forces and foot pronation: a new paradigm. Clin J Sport Med 2001;11(1):2–9.
6. McPoil TG, Hunt GC. Evaluation and management of foot and ankle disorders: present problems and future directions. J Orthop Sports Phys Ther 1995;21(6):381–8.
7. Harradine P, Gates L, Bowen C. If it doesn't work, why do we still do it? The continuing use of subtalar joint neutral theory in the face of overpowering critical research. J Orthop Sports Phys Ther 2018;48(3):130–2.
8. Jarvis HL, Nester CJ, Bowden PD, et al. Challenging the foundations of the clinical model of foot function: further evidence that the root model assessments fail to appropriately classify foot function. J Foot Ankle Res 2017;10(1):7.
9. Van Gheluwe B, Kirby KA, Roosen P, et al. Reliability and accuracy of biomechanical measurements of the lower extremities. J Am Podiatr Med Assoc 2002;92(6):317–26.
10. LaPointe SJ, Peebles C, Nakra A, et al. The reliability of clinical and caliper-based calcaneal bisection measurements. J Am Podiatr Med Assoc 2001;91(3):121–6.
11. Jarvis HL, Nester CJ, Jones RK, et al. Inter-assessor reliability of practice based biomechanical assessment of the foot and ankle. J Foot Ankle Res 2012;5(1):14.
12. Elveru RA, Rothstein JM, Lamb RL. Goniometric reliability in a clinical setting: subtalar and ankle joint measurements. Phys Ther 1988;68(5):672–7.
13. Kirby KA. What a recent study gets right and wrong about root biomechanics. Pod Today 2017;30(6). Available at: https://www.podiatrytoday.com/what-recent-study-gets-right-and-wrong-about-root-biomechanics. Accessed April 8, 2019.
14. Burssens A, Van Herzele E, Leenders T, et al. Weightbearing CT in normal hindfoot alignment—Presence of a constitutional valgus? Foot Ankle Surg 2018; 24(3):213–8.
15. Conti MS, Ellis SJ, Chan JY, et al. Optimal position of the heel following reconstruction of the stage II adult-acquired flatfoot deformity. Foot Ankle Int 2015; 36(8):919–27.
16. Frigg A, Nigg B, Davis E, et al. Does alignment in the hindfoot radiograph influence dynamic foot-floor pressures in ankle and tibiotalocalcaneal fusion? Clin Orthop Relat Res 2010;468(12):3362–70.
17. Gatt A, De Giorgio S, Chockalingam N, et al. A pilot investigation into the relationship between static diagnosis of ankle equinus and dynamic ankle and foot dorsiflexion during stance phase of gait: time to revisit theory? Foot 2017;30:47–52.

18. Dayton P, Feilmeier M, Parker K, et al. Experimental comparison of the clinical measurement of ankle joint dorsiflexion and radiographic Tibiotalar position. J Foot Ankle Surg 2017;56(5):1036–40.

19. Thordarson DB, Schmotzer H, Chon J, et al. Dynamic support of the human longitudinal arch. A biomechanical evaluation. Clin Orthop Relat Res 1995;316: 165–72.

20. Johnson CH, Christensen JC. Biomechanics of the first ray part I. The effects of peroneus longus function: a three-dimensional kinematic study on a cadaver model. J Foot Ankle Surg 1999;38(5):313–21.

21. Johnson CH, Christensen JC. Biomechanics of the first ray part V: the effect of equinus deformity: a 3-dimensional kinematic study on a cadaver model. J Foot Ankle Surg 2005;44(2):114–20.

22. Amis J. The split second effect: the mechanism of how equinus can damage the human foot and ankle. Front Surg 2016;3:38.

23. Ling JS, Ross KA, Hannon CP, et al. A plantar closing wedge osteotomy of the medial cuneiform for residual forefoot supination in flatfoot reconstruction. Foot Ankle Int 2013;34(9):1221–6.

24. Jordan TH, Rush SM, Hamilton GA, et al. Radiographic outcomes of adult acquired flatfoot corrected by medial column arthrodesis with or without a medializing calcaneal osteotomy. J Foot Ankle Surg 2011;50(2):176–81.

25. Kunas GC, Do HT, Aiyer A, et al. Contribution of medial cuneiform osteotomy to correction of longitudinal arch collapse in stage IIb adult-acquired flatfoot deformity. Foot Ankle Int 2018;39(8):885–93.

26. Ward CM, Dolan LA, Bennett DL, et al. Long-term results of reconstruction for treatment of a flexible cavovarus foot in Charcot-Marie-Tooth disease. J Bone Joint Surg Am 2008;90(12):2631–42.

27. Zhang JY, Du JY, Chen B, et al. Correlation between three-dimensional medial longitudinal arch joint complex mobility and medial arch angle in stage II posterior tibial tendon dysfunction. Foot Ankle Surg 2018. https://doi.org/10.1016/j. fas.2018.08.011.

28. Miniaci-Coxhead SL, Weisenthal B, Ketz JP, et al. Incidence and radiographic predictors of valgus tibiotalar tilt after hindfoot fusion. Foot Ankle Int 2017; 38(5):519–25.

29. Roukis TS. Metatarsus primus elevatus in hallux rigidus: fact or fiction? J Am Podiatr Med Assoc 2005;95(3):221–8.

30. Stevens J, Meijer K, Bijnens W, et al. Gait analysis of foot compensation after arthrodesis of the first metatarsophalangeal joint. Foot Ankle Int 2017;38(2): 181–91.

31. Hoppenfeld S. Physical exam of the spine & extremities. Norwalk (CT): Appleton & Lange; 1976.

32. Leetun DT, Ireland ML, Willson JD, et al. Core stability measures as risk factors for lower extremity injury in athletes. Med Sci Sports Exerc 2004;36(6):926–34.

33. Bakken A, Targett S, Bere T, et al. Muscle strength is a poor screening test for predicting lower extremity injuries in professional male soccer players: a 2-year prospective cohort study. Am J Sports Med 2018;46(6):1481–91.

34. Hreljac A, Marshall RN, Hume PA. Evaluation of lower extremity overuse injury potential in runners. Med Sci Sports Med 2000;32(9):1635–41.

35. Messier SP, Martin DF, Mihalko SL, et al. A 2-year prospective cohort study of overuse running injuries: the runners and injury longitudinal study (TRAILS). Am J Sports Med 2018;46(9):2211–21.

36. Willems TM, Witrouw E, De Cock A, et al. Gait-related risk factors for exercise-related lower-leg pain during shod running. Med Sci Sports Exerc 2007;39(2): 330–9.
37. Korpelainen R, Orava S, Karpakka J, et al. Risk factors for recurrent stress fractures in athletes. Am J Sports Med 2001;29(3):304–10.
38. Bennell KL. Risk factors for stress fractures in track and field athletes: a twelve-month prospective study. Am J Sports Med 1996;24(6):810–8.
39. Pelletier-Galarneau M, Martineau P, Gaudreault M, et al. Review of running injuries of the foot and ankle: clinical presentation and SPECT-CT imaging patterns. Am J Nucl Med Mol Imaging 2015;5(4):305–16.
40. Di Caprio F, Buda R, Mosca M, et al. Foot and lower limb diseases in runners: assessment of risk factors. J Sports Sci Med 2010;9:587–96.
41. Van der Worp H, Vrielink JW, Bredeweg SW. Do runners who suffer injuries have higher vertical ground reaction forces than those who remain injury-free? A systematic review and meta-analysis. Br J Sports Med 2016;50:450–7.
42. Engebretsen AH, Myklebust G, Holme I, et al. Intrinsic factors for groin injuries among male soccer players: a prospective cohort study. Am J Sports Med 2010; 38(10):2051–7.
43. Kaufman KR, Brodine SK, Shaffer RA, et al. The effect of foot structure and range of motion on musculoskeletal overuse injuries. Am J Sports Med 1999; 27(5):585–93.
44. Yates B. Chapter 16 - management of the sports patient. In: Turner WA, Merriman LM, editors. Clinical skills in treating the foot. Philadelphia: Elsevier; 2005. p. 393–430.
45. Liu H, Garrett WE, Moorman CT, et al. Injury rate, mechanism, and risk factors of hamstring strain injuries in sports: a review of the literature. J Sport Health Sci 2012;1:92–101.
46. Cabello EN, Hernandez DC, Marquez GT, et al. A review of risk factors for hamstring injury in soccer: a biomechanical approach. Eur J Hum Movement 2015;34:52–74.
47. Mills M, Frank B, Goto S, et al. Effect of restricted hip flexor muscle length on hip extensor muscle activity and lower extremity biomechanics in college-aged female soccer players. Int J Sports Phys Ther 2015;10(7):946–54.
48. Van Dyk N, Farooq A, Bahr R, et al. Hamstring and ankle flexibility deficits are weak risk factors for hamstring injury in professional soccer players: a prospective cohort study of 438 players including 78 injuries. Am J Sports Med 2018; 46(9):2203–10.
49. Ernlund L, de Almeida Vieira L. Hamstring injuries: update article. Rev Bras Ortop 2017;52(4):373–82.
50. Prior M, Guerin M, Grimmer K. An evidence-based approach to hamstring strain injury: a systematic review of the literature. Sports Med 2009;1(2):154–64.
51. Orchard J, Marsden J, Lord S, et al. Preseason hamstring muscle weakness associated with hamstring muscle injury in australian footballers. Am J Sports Med 1997;25(1):81–5.
52. Croisier JL, Ganteaume S, Binet J, et al. Strength imbalances and prevention of hamstring injury in professional soccer players: a prospective study. Am J Sports Med 2008;36(8):1469–75.
53. Witvrouw E, Danneels L, Asselman P, et al. Muscle flexibility as a risk factor for developing muscle injuries in male professional soccer players: a prospective study. Am J Sports Med 2003;31(1):41–6.

54. Watsford ML, Murphy AJ, McLachlan KA, et al. A prospective study of the relationship between lower body stiffness and hamstring injury in professional australian rules footballers. Am J Sports Med 2010;38(10):2058–64.
55. Kee MJ, Reid SL, Elliott BC, et al. Running biomechanics and lower limb strength associated with prior hamstring injury. Med Sci Sports Exerc 2009; 41(10):1942–51.
56. Bourne MN, Opar DA, Williams MD, et al. Eccentric knee flexor strength and risk of hamstring injuries in rugby union: a prospective study. Am J Sports Med 2015;43(11):2663–70.
57. Aderem J, Louw QA. Biomechanical risk factors associated with iliotibial band syndrome in runners: a systematic review. BMC Musculoskelet Disord 2015; 16:1517–23.
58. Powers CM. The influence of abnormal hip mechanics on knee injury: a biomechanical perspective. J Orthop Sports Phys Ther 2010;40(2):42–51.
59. Ferber R, Noehren B, Hamill J, et al. Competitive female runners with a history of Iliotibial band syndrome demonstrate atypical hip and knee kinematics. J Orthop Sports Phys Ther 2010;40(2):52–8.
60. Noehren B, Davis I, Hamill J. ASB clinical biomechanics award winner 2006 prospective study of the biomechanical factors associated with Iliotibial band syndrome. Clin Biomech 2007;22:951–6.
61. Louw M, Deary C. The biomechanical variables involved in the aetiology of Iliotibial band syndrome in distance runners: a systematic review of the literature. Phys Ther Sport 2014;15(1):64–75.
62. Fredericson M, Wolf C. Iliotibial band syndrome in runners: innovations in treatment. Sports Med 2005;35(5):451–9.
63. Orchard JW, Fricker PA, Abud AT, et al. Biomechanics of Iliotibial band friction syndrome in runners. Am J Sports Med 1996;24(3):375–9.
64. Miller RH, Lowry JL, Meardon SA, et al. Lower extremity mechanics of Iliotibial band syndrome during an exhaustive run. Gait Posture 2007;26:407–13.
65. Zazulak BT, Hewett TE, Reeves NP, et al. The effects of core proprioception on knee injury: a prospective biomechanical-epidemiological study. Am J Sports Med 2007;35(3):368–73.
66. Zazulak BT, Hewett TE, Reeves NP, et al. Deficits in neuromuscular control of the trunk predict knee injury risk. Am J Sports Med 2007;35(7):1123–30.
67. Tran AA, Gatewood C, Harris AH, et al. The effect of foot landing position on biomechanical risk factors associated with anterior cruciate ligament injury. J Exp Orthop 2016;3:13.
68. Boling MC, Padua DA, Marshall SW, et al. A prospective investigation of biomechanical risk factors for patellofemoral pain syndrome: the joint undertaking to monitor and prevent ACL injury (JUMP-ACL) cohort. Am J Sports Med 2009; 37(11):2108–16.
69. Lankhorst NE, Bierma-Zeinstra SM, van Middelkoop M. Risk factors for patellofemoral pain syndrome: a systemic review. J Orthop Sports Phys Ther 2012; 42(2):81–94.
70. Lin CF, Liu H, Gros MT, et al. Biomechanical risk factors of non-contact ACL injuries: a stochastic biomechanical modeling study. J Sport Health Sci 2012;1: 36–42.
71. Myer GD, Ford KR, Khoury J, et al. Biomechanics laboratory-based prediction algorithm to identify female athletes with high knee loads that increase risk of ACL injury. Br J Sports Med 2011;45(4):245–52.

72. Hewett TE, Myer GD, Ford KR, et al. Biomechanical measures of neuromuscular control and valgus loading of the knee predict anterior cruciate ligament injury risk in female athletes: a prospective study. Am J Sports Med 2005;33(4): 492–501.

73. Fong CM, Blackburn JT, Norcross MF, et al. Ankle-dorsiflexion range of motion and landing biomechanics. J Athl Train 2011;46(1):5–10.

74. Mendonca LD, Ocarino JM, Bittencourt NFN, et al. Association of hip and foot factors with patellar tendinopathy (jumper's knee) in athletes. J Orthop Sports Phys Ther 2018;48(9):676–84.

75. Witvrouw E, Bellemans J, Lysens R, et al. Intrinsic risk factors for the development of patellar tendinitis in an athletic population: a two-year prospective study. Am J Sports Med 2001;29(2):190–5.

76. Kannus VPA. Evaluation of abnormal biomechanics of the foot and ankle in athletes. Br J Sports Med 1992;26(2):83–9.

77. Alvarez-Nemegyei J. Risk factors for pes anserinus tendinitis/bursitis syndrome: a case control study. J Clin Rheumatol 2007;13(2):63–5.

78. Callahan LR. In: Fields KB, Grayzel J, editors. Overview of running injuries of the lower extremity. Waltham (MA): UpToDate inc; 2019. p. 1–25.

79. Fullem BW. Overuse lower extremity injuries in sports. Clin Podiatr Med Surg 2015;32(2):239–51.

80. Bennett JE, Reinking MF, Pluemer B, et al. Factors contributing to the development of medial tibial stress syndrome in high school runners. J Orthop Sports Phys Ther 2001;31(9):504–10.

81. Raissi GR, Cherati AD, Mansoori KD, et al. The relationship between lower extremity alignment and medial tibial stress syndrome among non-professional athletes. Sports Med Arthrosc Rehabil Ther Technol 2009;1(11):1–8.

82. Yates B, White S. The incidence and risk factors in the development of medial tibial stress syndrome among naval recruits. Am J Sports Med 2004;32(3): 772–80.

83. Sharma J, Golby J, Greeves J, et al. Biomechanical and lifestyle risk factors for medial tibia stress syndrome in army recruits: a prospective study. Gait Posture 2011;33:361–5.

84. Reinking MF. Exercise-related leg pain in female collegiate athletes: the influence of intrinsic and extrinsic factors. Am J Sports Med 2006;34(9):1500–7.

85. Munteanu SE, Barton CJ. Lower limb biomechanics during running in individuals with achilles tendinopathy: a systematic review. J Foot Ankle Res 2011; 4:15.

86. Mahieu NN, Witrouw E, Stevens V, et al. Intrinsic risk factors for the development of achilles tendon overuse injury: a prospective study. Am J Sports Med 2006; 34(2):226–35.

87. O'Neill S, Watson PJ, Barry S. A Delphi study of risk factors for achilles tendinopathy- opinions of world tendon experts. Int J Sports Phys Ther 2016;11(5): 684–97.

88. O'Neill S, Watson P, Barry S. 75 Plantarflexor muscle power deficits in runners with achilles tendinopathy. Br J Sports Med 2014;48(2):A49.

89. Lorimer AV, Hume PA. Achilles tendon injury risk factors associated with running. Sports Med 2014;44(10):1459–72.

90. Huang PY, Chen WL, Lin CF, et al. Lower extremity biomechanics in athletes with ankle instability after a 6-week integrated training program. J Athl Train 2014; 49(2):163–72.

91. Willems TM, Witrouw E, Delbaere K, et al. Intrinsic risk factors for inversion ankle sprains in male subjects: a prospective study. Am J Sports Med 2005;33(3): 415–23.

92. De Ridder R, Witrouw E, Dolphens M, et al. Hip strength as an intrinsic risk factor for lateral ankle sprains in youth soccer players: a 3-season prospective study. Am J Sports Med 2016;45(2):410–6.

93. Baumhauer JF, Alosa DM, Renstrom AF, et al. A prospective study of ankle injury risk factors. Am J Sports Med 1995;23(5):564–70.

94. Willems TM, Witrouw E, Delbaere K, et al. Intrinsic risk factors for inversion ankle sprains in females: a prospective study. Scand J Med Sci Sports 2005;15(5): 336–45.

95. Willems T, Witrouw E, Delbaere K, et al. Relationship between gait biomechanics and inversion sprains: a prospective study of risk factors. Gait Posture 2005; 21(4):379–87.

96. Beeson P. Posterior tibial tendinopathy: what are the risk factors? J Am Podiatr Med Assoc 2014;104(5):455–67.

97. Rabbito M, Pohl MB, Humble N, et al. Biomechanical and clinical factors related to stage I posterior tibial tendon dysfunction. J Orthop Sports Phys Ther 2011; 41(10):776–84.

98. Neville C, Flemister AS, Houck JR. Deep posterior compartment strength and foot kinematics in subjects with stage II posterior tibial tendon dysfunction. Foot Ankle Int 2010;31(4):320–8.

99. Raikin SM, Slenker N, Ratigan B. The association of a varus hindfoot and fracture of the fifth metatarsal metadiaphyseal junction: the jones fracture. Am J Sports Med 2008;36(7):1367–72.

100. Beeson P. Plantar fasciopathy: revisiting the risk factors. Foot Ankle Surg 2014; 20(3):160–5.

101. Riddle DL, Pulisic M, Pidcoe P, et al. Risk factors for plantar fasciitis: a matched case-control study. J Bone Joint Surg 2003;85(5):872–7.

102. Pohl MB, Hamill J, Davis IS. Biomechanical and anatomic factors associated with a history of plantar fasciitis in female runners. Clin J Sport Med 2009; 19(5):372–6.

103. Patel A, DiGiovanni B. Association between plantar fasciitis and isolated contracture of the gastrocnemius. Foot Ankle Int 2011;32(1):5–8.

104. Nakale NT, Strydom A, Saragas NP, et al. Association between plantar fasciitis and isolated gastrocnemius tightness. Foot Ankle Int 2018;39(3):271–7.

105. McNamee MJ. Analysis of plantar fasciitis risk factors among intercollegiate and recreational runners: a matched case-control study. Thesis submitted to the Graduate Council of Texas State University; 2016. p. 1–46.

106. Yoho RM, Carrington S, Dix B, et al. The association of metatarsus adductus to the proximal fifth metatarsal Jones fracture. J Foot Ankle Surg 2012;51(6): 739–42.

107. Fleischer AE, Stack R, Klein EE, et al. Forefoot adduction is a risk factor for Jones fracture. J Foot Ankle Surg 2017;56(5):917–21.

108. Becker J, James S, Wayner R, et al. Biomechanical factors associated with Achilles tendinopathy and medial tibial stress syndrome in runners. Am J Sports Med 2017;45(11):2614–21.

109. Jarvinen TA, Kannus P, Maffuli N, et al. Achilles tendon disorders: etiology and epidemiology. Foot Ankle Clin 2005;10(2):255–66.

110. Valmassy RL. Clinical biomechanics of the lower extremities. 1st edition. St. Louis (MO): Mosby; 1995.

Moving?

Make sure your subscription moves with you!

To notify us of your new address, find your **Clinics Account Number** (located on your mailing label above your name), and contact customer service at:

Email: journalscustomerservice-usa@elsevier.com

800-654-2452 (subscribers in the U.S. & Canada)
314-447-8871 (subscribers outside of the U.S. & Canada)

Fax number: 314-447-8029

Elsevier Health Sciences Division
Subscription Customer Service
3251 Riverport Lane
Maryland Heights, MO 63043

*To ensure uninterrupted delivery of your subscription, please notify us at least 4 weeks in advance of move.